Pregnancy Guide for First-Time Dads:

Understand the Pregnancy Stages, Become the Supportive Husband, Overcome Emotional Challenges, and Be the Father You Want to Be!!!

Taylor Anthony

MAI Digital Publishing

Copyright © 2024 by Taylor Anthony

All rights reserved.

The content contained within this book may not be reproduced, duplicated or transmitted without direct written permission from the author or the publisher.

Under no circumstances will any blame or legal responsibility be held against the publisher, or author, for any damages, reparation, or monetary loss due to the information contained within this book, either directly or indirectly.

Legal Notice:

This book is copyright protected. It is only for personal use. You cannot amend, distribute, sell, use, quote or paraphrase any part, or the content within this book, without the consent of the author or publisher.

Disclaimer Notice:

Please note the information contained within this document is for educational and entertainment purposes only. All effort has been executed to present accurate, up to date, reliable, complete information. No warranties of any kind are declared or implied. Readers acknowledge that the author is not engaged in the rendering of legal, financial, medical or professional advice. The content within this book has been derived from various sources. Please consult a licensed professional before attempting any techniques outlined in this book.

By reading this document, the reader agrees that under no circumstances is the author responsible for any losses, direct or indirect, that are incurred as a result of the use of the information contained within this document, including, but not limited to, errors, omissions, or inaccuracies.

Contents

Dedication	V
Introduction	VII
1. First-Time Fatherhood - The Three-Act Play	2
2. Mood Swings and Dad Things - Surviving the Emotional Twisters of Pregnancy	33
3. The Dad, the Doc, and the Baby Bump - Tackling the Healthcare Labyrinth	52
4. Navigating Nausea - Making Queasy Easy for First-Time Dads	75
5. The Home Stretch - When She Waddles, You Hustle	95
Dads Helping Dads	120
6. Embrace the Chaos - A Newbie's Guide to Unpredictable Joys of Fatherhood	123
7. Keep Calm and Daddy On - Surviving the Emotional Rapids of the Postpartum Period	144

8.	Dad by Day, Superhero by Night - Fatherhood in the 21st Century	163
9.	Coffee, Conference Calls, and Cuddles - The Modern Dad's Trifecta	183
10.	Womb Whisperer - My Journey to Becoming Baby's First Friend	204
11.	Surviving Baby Boot Camp - Becoming a Pro Dad	215

Conclusion	247
Afterword	251
Glossary	254
References	262

This book is dedicated to my beautiful wife Sofia and our two amazing boys Luca and Marco. Thank you for being my dream come true. Love Dad.

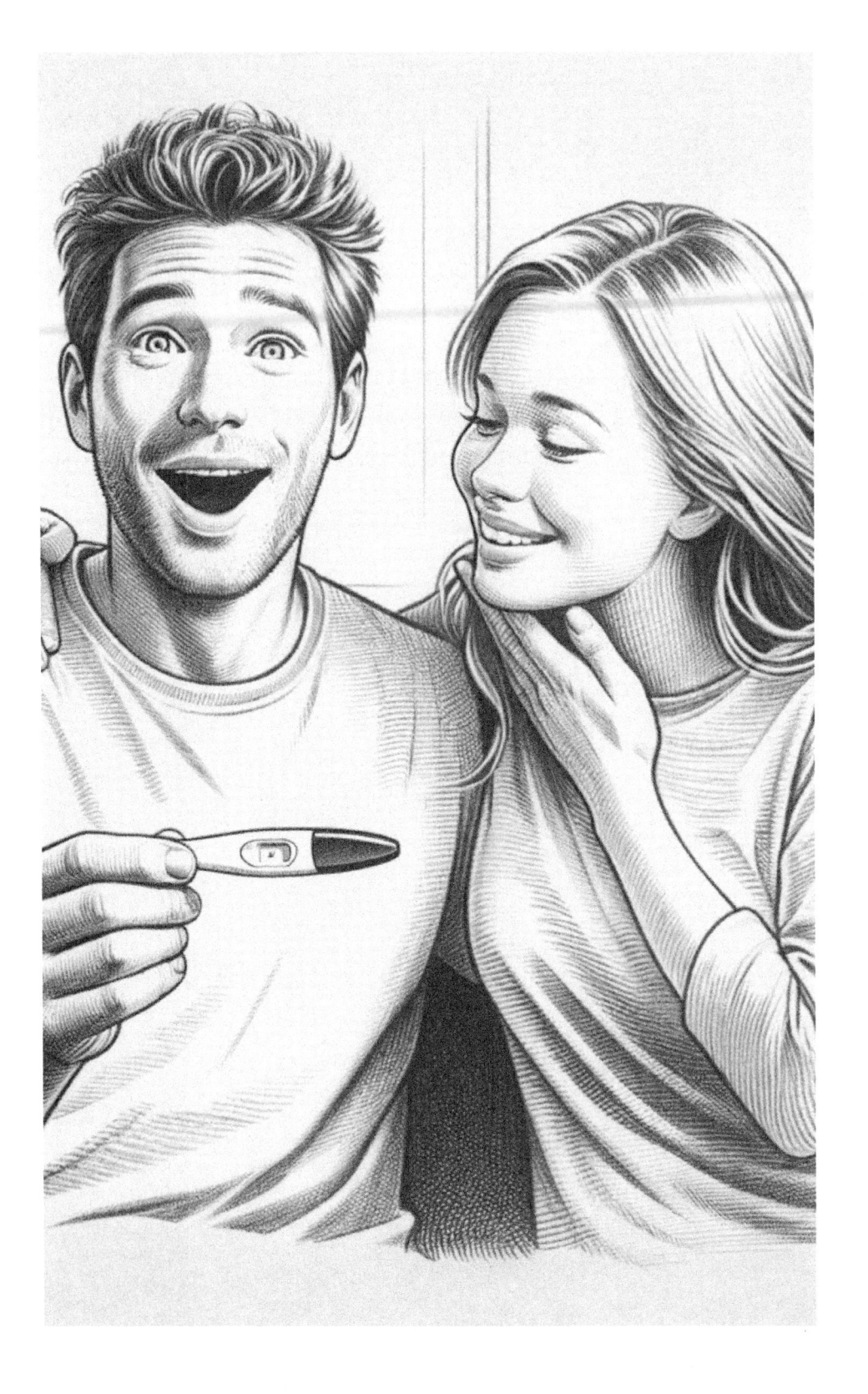

Introduction

Hey there, new dad! Congratulations on starting your exciting journey! Now, If your partner is already pregnant, double congratulations! And if you are both going for it, we're rooting for you! With that said, let's talk about your job responsibilities without delay.

On the bright side, feeling happiness and anticipation are your secondary tasks. What are your primary tasks? Your primary tasks include feeling inadequate and having self-doubt. Think of it as a full-time job with a 24/7 on-call schedule! But hey, don't worry! Millions of dads (including me!) have successfully made it through this, so you are in good company.

Now, first of all, don't beat yourself up if your mind is racing with questions. That's totally normal. In fact, it's daddy normal!

Wondering how to manage yourself mentally, physically, spiritually, emotionally, and financially as a first-time dad is all part of the daddy norm. You can even add a touch of "What in the world I have gotten myself into?" in that daddy normal. Trust me, you are not alone in feeling these things, my friend. It's as normal as mistaking the front of a diaper for the back in a sleep-deprived state (yep!). To put it into perspective, being a first-time dad is like experiencing anything important for the first time.

Remember the first time you hopped on a bicycle, the first day at a new job, or even the first day of marriage? You were a mix of many emotions at that time, but now you can advise anyone on navigating those experiences. Well, *daddyhood* is a bit like that. The first thing you need to do is to take care of your mental health.

Your mental health is your best tool in the shed—you need it working to handle the changes in your schedule, finances, and spouse. Without prioritizing your own well-being, nothing will get done.

Trust me: Your spouse will be going through a whirlwind crazier than you have ever seen—from morning sickness that feels like she took the wrong amusement park ride, mood swings that make it seem like she developed split personalities, to physical discomforts that may have her thinking she needs a hospital checkup every day. You need good mental health to handle all that.

Since your mental health is important as a dad, let's list some questions that are likely bouncing around in your head and making you restless. *Can I do things correctly? What kind of dad do I need to be? What if I make mistakes?* Take a deep breath, my friend. Those questions will stay confusing for some time, just like the first time you attempted to assemble a LEGO puzzle or IKEA furniture—with time and practice, you will master them. Eventually, you will see that life as a parent is a continuing education experience, filled with many new quandaries, questions, and quorums, over time in each new phase.

Let's start with the root of these questions, the one occupying most daddies' minds. It's imagining how to be the super-dads who have figured out life like a boss. The dads who can juggle work, family, and hobbies, and can probably even make dinner for everyone while lulling the baby. You may have seen some dads like that in your personal life, which made you nervous. But there's a secret they probably never let you realize: They often start someplace as confused as you.

The cooking process that made super-dads what they are contained a little love, a sprinkle of patience, and many trials and errors. Did they make mistakes? Oh yes. Did they repeat those mistakes? No (ignoring when they were sleep-deprived!). You can do that as well. Frank Pittman (n.d.) said something that rings true: "The end product of child-raising is not the child but the parent."

Who am I to say this regarding your journey? To answer that, I need you to imagine this: You are standing at the edge of an adventure, the adventure of fatherhood. The kind of adventure where you are given a quest to keep a tiny human being (plus their mother) alive and happy. Guess what? I have been on that roller-coaster, and I have got your back.

This book is there to teach you many things, but it's not just an information overload—it's where a conversation happens between an experienced dad and a new dad.

It's where an experienced dad opens up to a newer dad about his insights and stories: Where he messed up, what he did right, and what he learned from others in his daddy adventure. I have been in those sleep-deprived shoes before, wondering what that baby cry means. I have been in a position where I had to manage my and my spouse's mental health. Sometimes, I felt proud, sometimes, I felt anxious, and sometimes, I felt amazed. There's much more to these experiences, and this book gives you the necessary tools to go through this journey, fellow dad.

But before you dive into the insights contained in this book, I need you to gather some physical tools: pens, pencils, highlighters, and bookmarks. Scribble down your thoughts, highlight resonating bits, or dog-ear pages to which you would like to return. There's even a small notes section after each chapter and an extended glossary at the end, so jot a few notes down and look a few terms up. Whatever helps you absorb, apply, and remember rocks. This will come in handy later when the baby general is impatient with their orders, your mind clock is not registering what day of the month (and pregnancy stage!) it is, and you need reminders of what to do. Now, enjoy the journey and show that baby who's the dad.

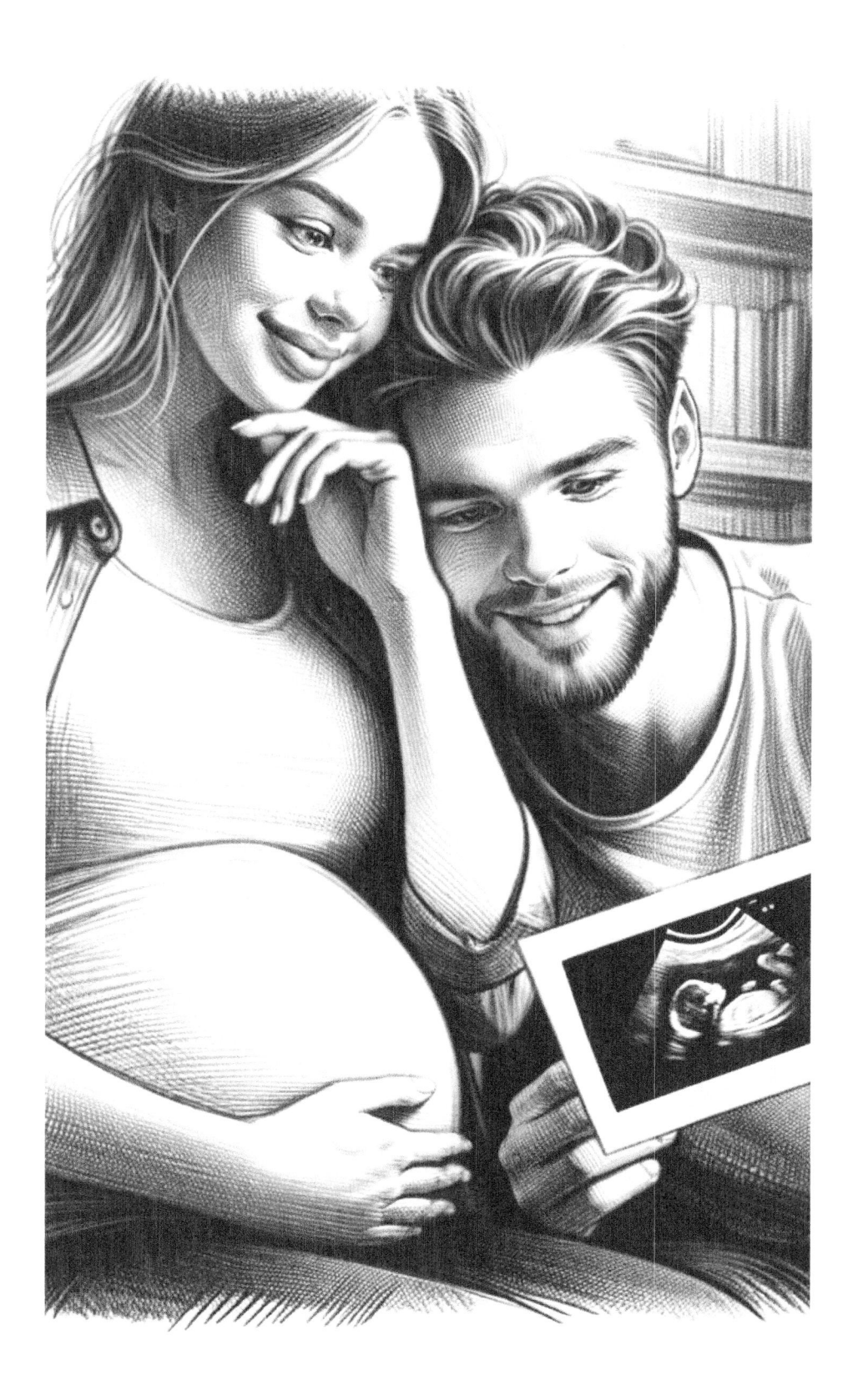

Chapter One

First-Time Fatherhood - The Three-Act Play

"A happy family is a reflection of a good father and a loving husband."

— Unknown

Parenting is a bit like learning your lines for a play. The more you prepare, the smoother the performance. This chapter is about equipping you with the required know-how of stages of pregnancy and the changes in them so that you can simulate them often. Therefore, put on your daddy suit for the play and get ready to roll!

THE BEGINNING OF THE THREE-ACT PLAY

It will be a three-act play (three trimesters) with a great ending. The 3 acts will take around 40 weeks to complete, with the timeline taking almost 12–14 weeks for each act.

Discovering the First Act

It's a game of cat and mouse to find out when the first act started. Updating your daddy encyclopedia, vomit is not the first sign that the first act has begun. It can take about 5–6 weeks for vomiting to happen.

It's a daddy's joy to find the pregnancy as soon as possible. Doing that in the first 2 weeks of the first act is the most difficult, as no significant change happens. But a dad can fight the odds by encouraging his spouse to share if she feels any different. Women's gut instinct can be somewhat accurate! But the sad thing is the odds are still stacked against the dad. The more precise signs are that your spouse has the following symptoms (Holland, 2023):

- missed period
- unusually high body temperature
- abnormal fatigue continuing for weeks
- changes to the breasts (e.g., swollen or tender)
- intense and frequent mood swings (e.g., anxiety, happiness, irritability, and sadness) coming and going like

- wind

- morning sickness

- increased need for urination

- stomach problems (e.g., constipation and bloating)

Noticeable signs like these happen 4-6 weeks into pregnancy. Missing her period is an excellent indicator of pregnancy, but by that point, you are already over 4 weeks into the first act—a little late find, but still good.

The first pregnancy test is taken at home using a pregnancy test device (shop that online). The pregnancy test can tell you the result when your wife is around 5-6 weeks into the pregnancy. If you found out before that, you get a daddy accolade. If you did not, now you know. In your excitement, you may think it's time to get to the doctor. Well, you are right!

Joining the Exciting Daddy Club

After confirming the pregnancy through a blood test at the hospital, it's about time to announce your presence to the local dad communities or online—if you haven't already done so. They will remain a source of mental and emotional support, and you can freely have conversations reserved for daddies there. Why am I mentioning this? Read on, and you will find out soon.

Sex Is Totally Okay

Hey, new dads! So, here's the deal: When you find out about the pregnancy, you don't have to go all monk mode and cut off sex from your life. The good news is, you can still have fun in the bedroom! Just remember, it's all about making sure your partner feels comfortable in whatever position you choose. And don't worry, it won't cause any complications! So, go ahead, keep the spark alive, and enjoy this exciting journey together!

Note:

The doctor might recommend abstinence later in the pregnancy, but they rarely do.

GUIDELINES TO FOLLOW IN THE THREE-ACT PLAY

The Training of the Heroine

Like female superheroes in movies, our heroine must also be physically and mentally strong. It doesn't take a dad-brain to realize that a healthier woman is better suited for childbirth. Doing physical exercises to stay fit is one of the best weapons in the heroine's arsenal in this play. Doctors recommend baby-friendly exercises even during pregnancy; being fit before pregnancy prepares the spouse to adjust better to the exercises and pregnancy.

The Supporting Cast in the Play

Food will be your spouse's supporting cast in this three-act play. Your spouse's food requirements will shoot through the roofs throughout Acts 2 and 3. The nutrients increase the size of breasts, uterus, blood volume, fat stores, and other crucial areas by a few pounds each. The resultant weight is massive—no kidding. She may gain 35 lb (16 kg) or more in just the last 6 pregnancy months! Take deep breaths and let that settle in. Digested that? Let's proceed.

The recommended weight increase for different body mass indexes (BMIs) by medical research is (Rasmussen et al., 2009):

- 28 to 40 lb below a BMI of 18
- 25 to 35 lb between a BMI of 18 to 24.9
- 15 to 25 lb between a BMI of 25 to 29.9
- 11 to 20 lb above BMI of 30

Before telling your spouse, think about how you can present this information so that your spouse doesn't have a mental meltdown—a challenging quest on the dad journey. Maybe mixing in that she only needs an extra 2–4 lb in the first 3 months if her BMI is healthy might help—probably not (Lindberg, 2020).

You both must know that eating handsomely will be the norm in the last two pregnancy stages.

Some monstrous urges of drinking alcohol (or smoking) may tempt your spouse because of the stress, but the dad has to step in firmly to stop those urges—the same is true for other unhealthy eating urges.

Now, let me pass you the ultimate daddy manual describing what your spouse should eat and what she shouldn't. You can bookmark this!

MAKING FOODS LIKE A CHEF

A healthy eating style for pregnancy is almost the same diet generally recommended by health professionals: eating complex carbs (avoiding simple carbs), healthy fats (avoiding unhealthy fats), lean protein, and taking a good dose of vitamins and minerals (Mayo Clinic Staff, 2022e).

Continuing my play analogy, there are five main supporting casts in the play:

- champion grains (whole grain bread, beans, legumes, and pasta)

- villainous treats (white bread, cookies, excess sugar, and chips)

- protein heroes (eggs, nuts, lean meat, fish, and chicken)

- veggie avengers (vegetables)
- fruitful dairies (fruits and milk)

Champion grains are your best bet at fighting against the villains. But champions alone are not enough to beat the villains—veggie avengers, protein heroes, and fruitful dairies are needed to support the champions.

Below are general tips when considering making a diet based on these things.

Adding Veggies to the Mix

It would help to create a menu considering how picky your spouse can be. All items on the menu for breakfast, lunch, and dinner should show the world that your wife is a pseudo-vegetarian. Veggies contain folic acid and many of the vitamins the spouse and baby require. Here is a daddy-styled menu to include veggies:

- For breakfast, mix veggies with eggs (half-fried or omelet).
- For lunch, veggie smoothies can be on the menu sometimes instead of fruit smoothies.
- For dinner, a simple salad with protein dishes.

Putting in Proteins and Fish

Proteins are crucial for the baby's growth, as Mayo Clinic has explained. Protein needs start their ascent to the roof from the beginning of the pregnancy. Those proteins will be used up, so Mama will fortunately (or unfortunately) not become a macho mama with them. Including the superheroes we mentioned earlier in the breakfast, lunch, and dinner helps to fill those needs. The good thing is that superheroes like eggs or fish (quite a number of fishes are rich in protein) and avengers like salads can aid each other at every mealtime.

Tip to Include the Above Foods in the Menu

Soup is a great tool in the daddy arsenal. Hot and delicious soups filled with veggies cut up by the daddy are a four-in-one package: Healthy, tasty, touching, and stomach-filling. The dad can shuffle multiple soups to give the tired spouse variety:

- soups with chicken and spinach
- tomato-based soups with onions and peppers
- soups with fish
- soups with cheese

And many more. Make sure to have multiple soupy options in the cabinet.

Champions Are Your Main Fighting Force

Heavyweight champions give Mama the nutrients (and the pounds) she needs. The champions need to be present in all meals in a heavy amount. It's easy to fall for the temptation of the villains and reduce the intake of champions, but the villains are lower fiber and nutritionally deficient. They can't compete against the champions!

The high fiber of whole grain foods is famous for preventing stomach problems like constipation. Champions like fortified cereals and legumes also give her different nutrients, such as folate, required for the development of different body parts of your baby. Just by taking the side of champions, you can reduce the chances of the baby developing a physical defect like spina bifida (Mayo Clinic Staff, 2022b). As they say, a person's company shapes the person—you also become a champion daddy by supporting the champions.

Adding Fruits and Milk

Calcium is necessary for the bone strength of both Baby and Mama, while fruits help prevent birth defects, as explained by Mayo Clinic Staff (2022b). Fruits and milk can be added in a supplementary way to meals, like eating apples or oranges an hour after breakfast or drinking a fruit shake at mealtime.

Tips to Include All Four Superpowers in the Menu

Some foods that include all these three things are:

- sandwiches made using whole grain bread, filled with chicken (or other lean proteins), and a lot of lovely veggies. A tasty spread can be used to give it a special daddy touch. Also, a glass of fruit shake can go well with this.

- soups made using beans and other legumes with the addition of meat and veggies. There are many combinations to last several pregnancies!

- whole grain pasta mixed with homemade vegetable sauces and the addition of meat. A fruit salad can be great with this.

- fortified whole grain cereals mixed with milk and everyone's favorite carrots (or other veggies). They are suitable for breakfast and can be taken alongside fruits.

Hey, that's all for food! I want to give you all the instructions from the cereal brand to the amount of milk you should add, but this is not a cookbook! The cookbooks and dad community can help you further on this topic. For now, we look at the supplements that go well with a healthy food lifestyle.

Stocking on Prenatal Vitamins

The heart, brain, and spine will be under development by week 4 (Marcin, 2017). Since we only get certified as new dads in the making after week 6 of pregnancy, we miss out on some critical baby development stages. If Mama's diet includes all sorts of strange things, this can easily hamper the growth of Dad's new star! That's unacceptable!

Now, there's good and bad news related to this. Let's first go with the good news to make our day! A mama hoping to be pregnant can adopt the healthy mama lifestyle (food, supplements, and exercise) before signs of pregnancy—which gets the baby all the nutrients they need when dear mama and papa are still in the dark about the new life. This is the whole background behind the quest to stock vitamins. The reward of the quest is successfully helping the baby develop throughout the pregnancy stages.

Hold on tight. It's time for the bad news! The mama has to keep to the vitamins and healthy diet with vigor and discipline resembling a devout worshiper all the time—before pregnancy signs and after them—and the dad has to be the watchman ensuring this happens! Talk about a tough job. Fight on, Daddy!

With that said, the recommended supplements are (Mayo Clinic Staff, 2022e)

- **High Priority**
  - folic acid
  - iron
  - calcium

- vitamin D

- **Others**
  - vitamin C
  - vitamin A
  - vitamin E
  - B vitamins
  - zinc
  - iodine

Folic acid and iron are needed for the baby's safe growth, while calcium and vitamin D help grow the baby's teeth and bones.

Additionally, Mama will need an omega-3 supplement if her diet doesn't include fish high in omega-3 fatty acids for any reason.

Minding the Side-Effects

There can be some side effects of consuming supplements. Mayo Clinic Staff (2023) says that a zinc overdose alone can cause issues like numbness and weakness in the arms as well as in the legs. Talk about being a nutrient with a lot of smack in it. Some are more dangerous—extra vitamin A can cause harm to your baby! *Pretty dangerous*. That's why it's a must not to overdose on any vitamin supplement.

The higher priority and lower priority division is just an attempt to divide by their vital role. It's better to consult the doctor for the recommended dosages, as your healthcare provider might suggest lower or higher doses of certain nutrients depending on the tests.

With the general guidelines clear (finally), let's continue to what happens after we find a baby intruder is coming into the house.

ACT 1: BIRTH OF A DADVENTURE

The first major signs and the pregnancy test already signal that the big game is about to start. However, the *dadventure* officially only begins after the doctor gives their approval. After the confirmation, the dad may want to stock extra food for the journey, but there's no need! Most women retain previous appetite or feel a decrease in it in the first act.

Why's that?

Firstly, the body only wants healthy food, not extra food. Another reason is that vomiting starts around week 5, remember? It continues for several weeks. No human would desire food in that state! That condition can make the mama especially tired and queasy—resulting in you having to clean up the gastro galaxy.

But, you can be happy knowing that research shows vomiting is a good sign for baby health, and you are making a noble sacrifice for the *babyland*! (Hinkle et al., 2016). The baby may not care about your sacrifice, but your spouse will appreciate it.

The dad in the dadventure will encounter several hurdles in the first act. Like a regular movie or act, many changes happen in the beginning to set the stage for what's to come next

Mama Changes in the First Act

Morning All-Day-And-Night Sickness

Commonly known as morning sickness, it doesn't only happen in the morning. It's more like that surprise twist in the movie plot. Mama will feel fine one moment and suddenly nauseous the next. Daddy can take supporting words or ginger tea out of the toolkit to help the mama in the unexpected scenario. It's natural for mama to have frequent bouts of morning sickness until the end of month 3 of pregnancy.

Fatigue That Doesn't Care About Anything

Morning sickness and fatigue also become partners of each other during pregnancy. Feeling queasy and vomiting is bound to make the mama tire just by itself. Still, more changes are happening that also contribute to fatigue: changes to breasts, increased heart rate, frequent trips to the washroom, stomach problems, and rising female hormone progesterone that supports female pregnancy all contribute to body fatigue.

I want to give you an analogy to help you feel what that can be like. Pregnancy can be like binge-watching a Netflix series, *Pregnancy: The Ultimate Marathon*, 24/7. Hopefully, there's no such series!

When the fatigue gets too much, the champion dad swoops in to save the day. He encourages mom to rest and sleep as much as needed, and cooks her favorite meals to brighten her appetite.

To fulfill the legacy of being a champion dad, he must up his game and know the best practices for increasing sleep quality. For instance, a cold, silent, dark room improves sleep quality. Additionally, exercise can also increase sleep quality.

Mood Swings

Mood swings are like the reveals of the play. It's like when the movie suddenly drops new information on you. Your spouse will be sharing all these new emotions she's experiencing. One moment, she will laugh and share positive thoughts; the next, she can burst into tears and share some not-so-positive thoughts. The hormones go on a roller-coaster, making her emotions go up and down on any given day. She will alternate moods between happiness, sadness, and anxiety from time to time.

Sometimes, she may have negative thoughts not because she genuinely thinks like that but because the hormone masterminds are making her think *that's what she thinks.* In all those moments, you need to be the understanding costar in the play—giving her the emotional anchor and positivity she needs.

As for things to avoid? Never, and I mean NEVER, mention that she's "acting hormonal." Trust me, that's a grenade you don't want to pull the pin on.

Healthy Training Routine

Health professionals recommend light exercises like walking and yoga. Heavy exercises of all forms are a no-no as they put an extra toll on the body (when there's already a lot to deal with). Light exercise helps with mood and sleep problems while preparing the body for the upcoming overload of pounds. Equally important, it's also better for the baby (American College of Obstetricians and Gynecologists, n.d.).

The duration of the exercises depends on the mom's fitness. If she wasn't invested in walking before, she can start with 10 minutes a day, 5 times a week—continuing up to 30 minutes daily.

Safety Tip!!!:

She should stay away from bad surfaces and rocky paths to avoid falling.

If Mama is more comfortable doing yoga, that's good, but she must avoid difficult yoga moves. Moves like abdomen twisters, backbends, hopping, headstands, and lying on your back (after week 20) must be avoided. The last one probably sounded *super weird*. That position can compress an important vein, reducing blood flow to your partner and the fetus (Cinelli, 2022). Talk about being scary! That's why it's better to consult a health professional about yoga positions before making them a staple exercise!

If your partner wants some alternative exercises, then Pilates, swimming, and stationary bike classes are safer options she can pick after consulting the dos and don'ts with a health professional.

Changes in Dad's Little Star

In the first act, Dad's little star develops some big parts: The brain, spinal cord, organs, vocal cords, kidneys, and heart (Marcin, 2017). Because these are crucial parts, the biggest fear of parents also has the highest chance of happening. After passing Act 1 safely, about 99 out of 100 pregnancies become safe from miscarriages, the source says. This means the risk becomes almost nonexistent.

Thankfully, the champion dad has done his best to ensure the baby's safety by ensuring that the mama is taking

- supplements and diet correctly before and after pregnancy signs.

- rest and avoid stress during the first act. The champion dad has given emotional support to the mama when needed.

- light exercise sessions of 30 minutes daily, 3–5 times a week.

Secret baby reveal:

The baby develops a heartbeat in the first trimester. According to Marcin (2017), the heartbeat starts high and rises from 100 beats per minute (bpm) around the 6th week to 150 bpm in the 9th week. Don't expect to notice it without an ultrasound, though. The good news is that the doctor usually suggests an ultrasound around the 12-week mark. Yay to that!

ACT 2: THE BELLY CHRONICLES – GROWING PAINS AND GAINS

In the middle of the play, the plot thickens! Mama's in the action movie part of her pregnancy. The heroine's body has started to adjust to the changes. Many previous unexplained plots like morning sickness get largely solved starting week 13, and she has a newfound energy boost. The heroine goes on many adventures (shopping sprees) to prepare for the coming showdown. Few changes happen in the second act, as the first act is where most things that set the stage for the three-act play have already happened.

Mama Changes in the Second Act

Some New Challengers in the Play

The heroine has solved many of the obstacles facing her before. Seeing that, some new villains will appear to annoy her on her journey. Some of the typical villains are villain leg cramps and villain heartburn. Also, increased appetite is the boss monster that has just shown his appearance and will stay until the end.

Body Weight Gain: The Real Challenger

All superheroes need to have a good amount of body weight! There was one thing similar in the recommended weight increase guidelines before—mama weight increases in all of them! Only the rate is different. Now, if Mama gained more or less than the 2–4 lb recommended (a little away from ideal), she should make up for it in this and the next trimester (Lindberg, 2020). Excluding that, the standard weight gain rate per week for different BMIs is (Rasmussen et al., 2009):

- "healthy": around 0.9 lb
- "underweight": slightly more than 1 lb
- "overweight": 0.5 lb

As a general rule, health professionals recommend around 350 extra calories for 1 lb of weight gain during the second trimester (Lindberg, 2020).

A little more than half of a healthy sandwich and a glass of skim milk may hit the 350 target recommended for a healthy BMI. Gaining too much weight per week than the recommended guidelines can make the baby bigger than average, causing problems at delivery for everyone! Gaining too little may make delivery timing earlier than desired. So, it's better to stick to recommended guidelines.

Tip:

The calorie gain rates I mentioned are averages. Don't let Mama starve herself, as some weeks can increase body requirements more than others. The overall target can be maintained if some weeks compensate for the weeks she eats extra.

Note:

Leg cramps and heartburn can also happen in the third trimester, so I have given details and tips for these 2 things as I discuss Act 3 in detail in Chapter 5.

Changes in Dad's Little Star

The baby starts urinating at the beginning of Act 2. The baby's maneuvers increase greatly in this act: they also start to urinate, suck, and kick! (Marcin, 2017).

The same source explains that their ear and eye development is enough that they may detect your voice and see lights in Mama's body around week 18. The ear development in week 20 is the next significant milestone—the baby can hear voices more clearly. It's time for the dad to pounce at the opportunity to make the first dad jokes he has in his arsenal.

It will help the baby recognize the dad's musical voice (fortunately, the baby can't negate the self-praise). Week 23 is the next milestone of Act 2: The baby starts showing his tae kwon do-style kicking moves.

Growing Gains of Act 2

Act 2 differs from Act 1 in that there are growing gains instead of only pains. The middle of the movie is the time to do things and enjoy the parent life. Some good stuff (pun alert!) that should be done in Act 2 are:

- teaching ethics to the baby starting week 18

- going on shopping sprees to stock up on baby gear: baby clothes, decorations for the nursery, baby bed, and other things discussed in Chapter 11

- investing in new equipment for Mama, like maternity wear and loose clothing

- feeling how much the baby has learned tae kwon do around week 23

- spreading the news of pregnancy to family and friends (your call!)

- thinking of baby names if you haven't done before already

Although Act 2 can be much more enjoyable for both parents than Act 1, Act 1 is also special as it brings new excitement. After Act 2, the dadventure proceeds toward its showdown, where a cute ending awaits.

ACT 3: DAD'S DEBUT – FROM BUMP TO BABY

Act 3 returns to a relatively serious tone as deserving of its fate as the showdown. Some new and old challenges team together to fight against the heroine. The baby's arrival is imminent, and the suspense causes the heroine and the hero to get super nervous (and equally excited).

Mama Changes in the Third Act

Body Weight Gain: Next Stage

The body weight gain becomes more robust in Act 3. For different BMIs, almost the same average weekly gain as of Act 1 is recommended. However, since the monster is stronger, instead of 350 calories, an extra 400–500 calories may be needed to gain the same weight for a healthy body. Think of it as a lot of energy is used in the showdown against the boss (to meet the increased energy requirements of the baby).

Tip:

As in Act 2, the exact weight gain guideline applies: Don't restrict Mama if she wants to eat more in some weeks.

The Aid of a Trusty Ally

Mama may experience mood swings, aches, and pains from time to time. The dependable daddy encourages a lot of rest and gives emotional support again using his dad jokes. After Dad, the next ally is the health professional. They take frequent tests to ensure the Mama and Baby duo's health never goes off track.

The Occupying Force Called Big Bump

A prominent occupying force called the big bump is visible on the mama as the belly protrudes rapidly. The occupying force is a big boss, blocking almost all travel routes. Travel restrictions take effect, and cruise ships and airlines put limitations. Cruise ships can often be strict regarding travel bans, while airlines may want you to have permission from a health professional.

If you are considering traveling, you should check the policies of the airline and cruise company you plan to use to see how the restrictions will affect your partner. These companies may have a policy of not letting second-trimester pregnant women travel.

The dad is also in the grasp of the occupying force and has to stay close to the mom. The occupying force is difficult to handle without prior preparations—the clothing prepared in advance in Act 2 helps a lot at this final boss stage.

Changes in Dad's Little Star: Final Form

Starting in week 25, the baby finally understands the importance of a chill break. Baby starts taking rest after being active, but that doesn't mean the baby will stop their activity (still a hard worker like daddy). Health professionals recommend telling if the movement feels less around week 27. The amount of tissue around the brain increases and then weight gain accelerates around week 35. By week 38, the baby almost reaches complete form.

The rough baby specifications will be 19 in. long and 7.5 lb heavy—not up for sale, though (Marchin, 2017). If the baby is born before completing 40 weeks, the baby can be a few inches smaller. The ending of the play is imminent any time at that point and usually happens around week 40—1 week, plus or minus.

Those are the main guidelines that I can tell you as a dad. There are some things that only the health professional can say to you, like the amount of supplement intake, ultrasound dates, test dates, and other situation-specific information. So, I have created a section on it separately so that it's easier to refer to later.

THE DOCTOR ALLY: HEALTH PROFESSIONAL

The doctor remains the much-needed instructor in the play who corrects any directional problems in the martial arts the hero and heroine practice. The heroine may have contacted this ally regarding dietary, medication, and supplement information before the pregnancy. Still, regarding the play's story, this ally only appears after the 6th week.

Encounters With the Doctor

The doctor will conduct a big examination consisting of many smaller tests to gauge the capacities of the heroine, ranging from supplement intake to travel and lifestyle guidelines.

Most guidelines stay the same: No smoking, no alcohol, healthy diet, and exercise. The tests taken by the doctor will give the fine-tuned calorie, supplement, and exercise requirements for the mama by seeing the BMI, body fitness, and other things in the test results.

Tip:

The doctor can't open your mind to know what's in it. It's best to be open about the questions and things you both think may be a problem. Past substance abuse, past domestic abuse, current lifestyle, and so on are things that your healthcare provider will take into account to provide your partner with a better plan.

Regular checks will happen after the first encounter with the doctor, like the weekly updates on your favorite show. The only difference is that regular checkups happen once a month in Act 1 to make for 1–2 more checkups before Act 2 starts. Then, checkups become bimonthly toward the end of Act 2 (around week 28) and will increase in importance and frequency toward the end of the play.

The list of tests and ultrasounds that the doctor will order as the mama goes through pregnancy is long, like the Wall of China, but those tests are a part of the standard operating procedures.

Just some of the things that are tested:

- blood type
- levels of iron and other nutrients
- previous vaccinations
- current infections
- specific disease tolerances

Depending on the test results, the doctor can decide what other tests Mama needs to take and how many supplements she needs. Instructions in each case can vary, and the health provider is in the best place to tell you all the dos and don'ts. In some cases, they may order an ultrasound at week 12, while in others, at week 7.

That's why I won't be going into details about the specific tests, as the doctor will tell you all the test reports you need to submit during regular checkups.

Finally, another congratulations, new dads! We have officially completed the crash course on the wild and wacky world of pregnancy. But we are still not done. This book is about to take you deeper into the thrilling roller-coaster ride of sleepless nights, diaper crises, and the occasional victory dance when you successfully calm your little one. Brace yourselves for this crazy adventure, and let's do it together!

Notes

PREGNANCY GUIDE FOR FIRST-TIME DADS

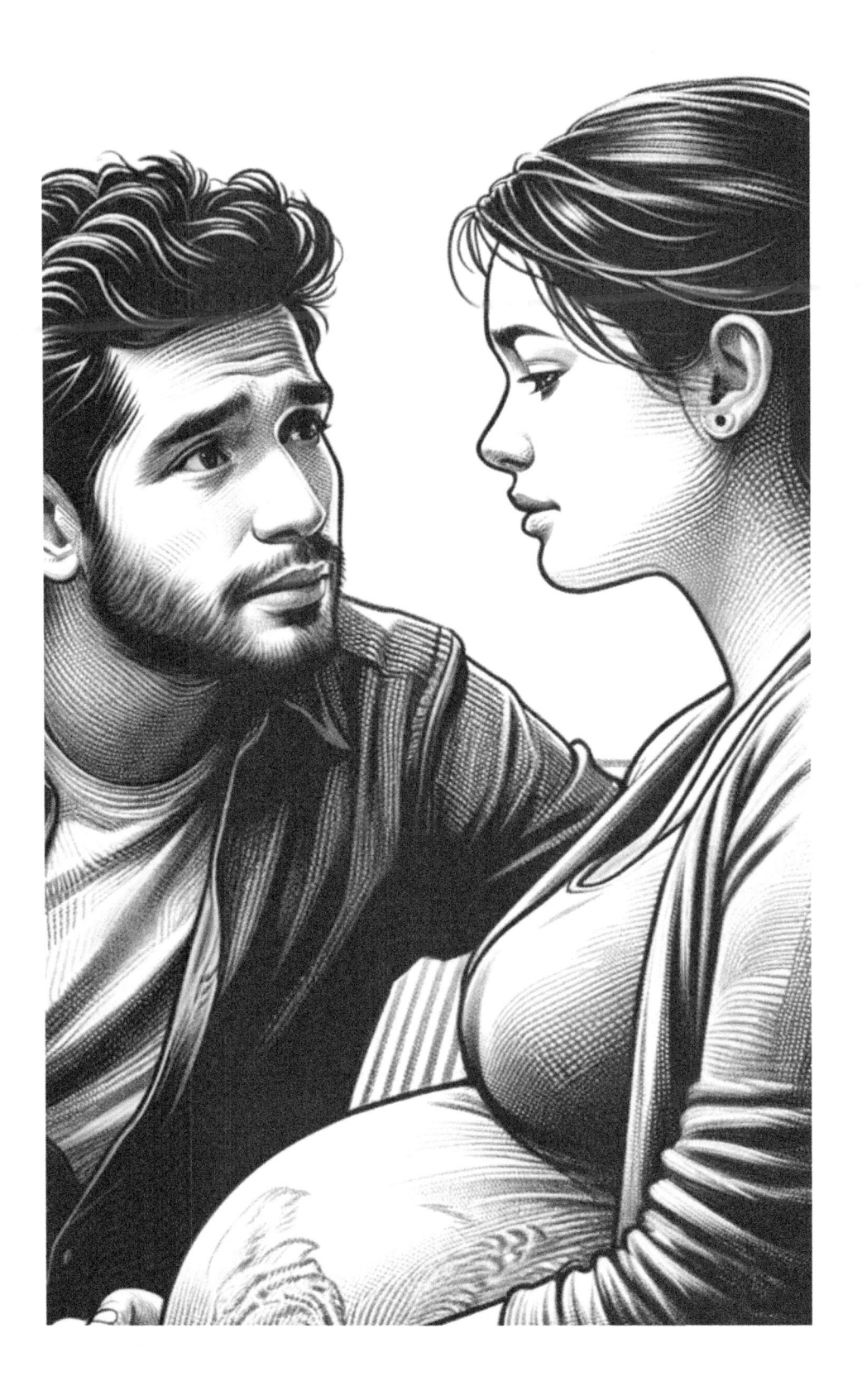

Chapter Two

Mood Swings and Dad Things - Surviving the Emotional Twisters of Pregnancy

"Empathy is a respectful understanding of what others are experiencing."
- Marshall B. Rosenberg

Mood swings are like a tiny fraction of the adventure, maybe just 5%–10%. But they can sneak up on you out of nowhere, leaving you scratching your head. However, fear not, new dads! The secret is to realize that Mama is experiencing mood swings.

Without this realization, you may be caught up in unexpected debates, which can strain your relationship. And hey, let's not forget, these debates aren't exactly great for anyone's health, especially not for the little one on the way. So, let's become the ultimate mood-swing detectors and crack the code behind these unpredictable mood swings in this chapter!

CRACKING THE CODE ON PREGNANCY HORMONES: WHAT'S BEHIND THOSE MOOD SWINGS

Mood swing. Sounds like a magic spell, right? Well, this magic spell isn't just for pregnancy. It happens to both boys and girls during their teenage years.

Now, let's take a trip down memory lane, my friend. Remember those wild things we did as a teenager when our hormones were all over the place? Well, guess what? Your spouse is all grown up now, so her mood swings will be a more adult version of that, with a few more factors at play.

Now, let me break it down for you and give you the inside scoop on what's causing those mood swings. That will help us know how we can navigate mood swings.

Brain Remodeling

Mama's brain goes through a brain renovation during pregnancy. It's like a construction crew has been hired to work on the brain. They prune away some brain stuff and her brain loses some volume. Sounds freakish? Brain experts say it's good for us (Hoekzema et al., 2022). Here's why.

The mama becomes an even better mama after the process. It's like her brain is rewiring to prioritize the child above other bucket list items. This means less preference for gatherings and more preference for the baby.

You may see her focusing more on baby decorations and all things baby: baby diapers, cribs, room, and so on. She will sit still one moment and then clean the baby's room in the next for the eighth time of the day. It's like a superhero transforming. Her body will transform into the ultimate mama mode, and she will do things like a pro.

Hormones at Their Full-Time Gig

Hormones are powerful. During pregnancy, they become extra active. It's like someone hired them for a full-time gig. Just remember how the male mind can become a little… distracted when it comes to mating. It should show you hormone power.

Women are also affected by a hormone party during pregnancy. Two big shots, estrogen and progesterone, lead the hormone party (Barth, 2023). To help understand them, let's break down their functions.

Estrogen

It's the in-house mood manager. It's associated with anxiety, irritability, feeling low, and so on. That's why when Mama goes through mood swings, estrogen is probably playing the DJ part, mixing things and riling everything up.

Progesterone

This hormone is all about keeping the body loose and chill. It helps loosen the muscles and joints. As this hormone's levels increase, and it starts working overtime, it takes payback by becoming a sneaky source of body fatigue.

The result of hormones responsible for mood regulation and body management having a party in the body is on another level. The increase of these hormones can turn any simple question like, "How was your day?" into a 3-hour crying fest. But don't worry, dad. Chalk it up to the hormones, and you will be less stressed. Remember, this is perfectly normal behavior when having mood swings.

Work Fatigue

Act 1 hits like a freight train, while Act 3 is like trying to climb Mount Everest with a big belly! Getting some z's becomes mission impossible, and your partner's body becomes jelly from all the exhaustion. And guess what? That fatigue comes with a bonus package: a tired mind and a bad mood. It's hard to keep those smiles on when running on an empty tank.

The Summer List of Worries

Your partner's worry list can contribute to mood swings a lot: There's the constant fear that nausea may strike at any moment in the first trimester, making even the most mundane tasks extra exhaustive. And let's not forget about the struggle with body image issues in the second and third trimesters—watching the belly grow within weeks is like witnessing something straight out of a sci-fi movie! Then there's the anxiety of being a new mother, with all the unknowns and the pressure to do everything right. And, of course, the worries about finances and the baby's health. But fear not, new dad!

In this chapter, we will dive into some listening techniques that will help you navigate through the worries, and in Chapter 7, we will explore a therapy technique that will aid in making those worries disappear faster than a magician's rabbit!

The Result

Considering the above, if you find your partner sobbing at a commercial one minute and then getting extremely mad over an empty ice cream container in the fridge the next, don't worry, it happens. She may suddenly resent you or her friends for enjoying a regular lifestyle, or she may be overjoyed that her belly is growing—that's just how mood swings work. To navigate this turbulence, my friend, effective communication is key. It's similar to sailing through a stormy sea; everyone must communicate well to keep the ship afloat.

EFFECTIVE COMMUNICATION: THE BRIDGE OVER TROUBLED WATER

Trying for effective communication during pregnancy is like trying to bathe a cat. You both are determined, but getting to the same page can take a while.

Your Blueprint

In pregnancy, the art of communication involves listening and feeling empathy. It's time to use our ears for more than just holding eyeglasses. The mission behind listening is to know when it's time to ask more questions versus when to say, "I feel you, Babe," even if you don't have a clue what she's getting at.

Showing Empathy

As a man, we can have a "barrier" when understanding what our partners are getting at. Our operating system features a priority matrix that works differently. So, it's no wonder that sometimes it may feel like she's fussing over nothing.

But here's the thing: Think about environmental conservationists. They may not directly experience the devastation caused by climate change, but they still work to protect ecosystems. They demonstrate empathy by acknowledging its impact on people living in other areas.

So, even if you don't understand why she's feeling something right now, trust that there must be a damn good reason behind it. It's important not to be a know-it-all. Don't go full-dismissive, even if you don't understand something at the moment.

Similarly, sometimes, it's just about letting her talk. Even if you don't fully understand, *be understanding* and give her the space to express herself.

Listening Actively

Basics of listening actively: When she's talking, don't just hear, listen. It's like catching a rare Pokémon—it needs your full attention. If your partner is talking, put down the controller or whatever you have in your hand (and mind) and focus on what she's saying. Go further by turning your body toward her and looking into her eyes. You need to make her feel you are just focused on her universe. It will keep you in her good books.

Your attention will fall like stones thrown, so reel it back. Asking a lot of questions shows you are interested and keeps you focused. And here's the secret: Genuinely care about how she's feeling physically and emotionally, and let her see that interest.

Navigating Overreactions

Sometimes, you may find yourself exasperated and wondering "*How can someone in the world do that*" when you encounter her

- overreactions.

- tantrums.

- melodramatic minutes.

It can be as simple as throwing a tantrum about some cravings, such as insisting on organic, gluten-free, dairy-free potato chips at 2 a.m. I remember one day during my wife's second trimester; she started crying out of the blue while watching a cereal commercial. The reason? "The Cheerios look so happy together," she sniffed. Yep, hormones can do that. Using a combination of listening and empathy will help us navigate such things with ease.

Combining Empathy and Active Listening

Let's look at how empathy and active listening can help us in everyday interactions.

Setting 1

You enter the bedroom and find your spouse crying.

What to do?

Ask her what's troubling her and listen. Maybe she's feeling insecure as a new mom or something similar. In that case, instead of fixing the problem, listen and validate her by telling her that what she's experiencing is normal.

Setting 2

You asked your partner for a meal, and she overreacted like you asked her to run a marathon.

Now, instead of letting that override your mind, see whether she needs support. Ask her if you can help her around with anything. Maybe there will be an outpour of emotions because she was feeling overwhelmed. Listen and offer understanding and support.

Setting 3

You just got up from bed, and the first thing you hear are harsh words from your spouse. Don't take her remarks personally; ask her if she needs help. Cook the morning meal or order it if you can. Listen to her concerns if she's willing to open up.

Setting 4

It's not uncommon for some serious forgetting to happen often during pregnancy.

So imagine this: You ask her to bring some bread from the store, and she comes back with dog food. The instructions were probably clear in her mind. It's just that they got overwritten somewhere along the way. Yes, totally not her fault!

Setting 5

Have you ever heard that couples start looking alike after spending years together? During pregnancy, they can even begin to sound like each other. You may ask her, "Where's the remote?" and a similar question may reflect. This kind of mind fog can happen, my friend. Sometimes, she may not have the capacity to process simple things.

As the above made it clear, adopt a listen-first, no-anger policy. Later in this chapter are some guiding principles to help you, but they all operate on this policy.

Tip:

It's best to listen thoroughly without overreacting. Otherwise, she may consciously/unconsciously omit certain things (including secret snack times) in the future because she knows you will overreact.

Note:

I would highly recommend reading a book on emotional intelligence.

Your Emotions Need a Response Too

Fellow dad-to-be, you also have to take care of yourself emotionally. Sometimes, there may be mood swings that make you frustrated and angry. Even if you realize they are mood swings and a small price to pay for becoming a dad, it's human nature to feel troubled when our emotional feathers are disturbed.

Handy Tip:

After listening, pick a good time to share your thoughts and feelings. A gentle and understanding tone is all you need to convey most things, even if they are somewhat unpleasant. You may even tell her that her breath smells bad, and she won't mind! When you don't know what tone to go by, go by the default gentle tone. It works wonders.

Cracking the Communication Problems

Communication problems can increase a lot during pregnancy. The hormones will crank up the volume of thoughts she could have ignored before.

She may beat herself up over whether she's eating right, drinking right, exercising enough, and so on. Things may be going good at one point, and you may feel she's alright, then a woman next door asks, "Wow, are you expecting twins?" leading to a new cycle of doubt regarding whether the belly is popping abnormally.

To handle this mixer of endless doubts, listening and empathy come to help. Listening helps us tune into her doubts and feelings at any moment. Empathy helps us think of ways to soothe her. These two things are your superpower as a dad.

Mama Community at the Rescue

You are a dad with superpowers, but you are still a dad at the end of the day. You can do your best, but resolving everything is impossible. Mama communities can be a help in those situations. They contain moms who can support and resolve her doubts in a way you never can. They can understand where she comes from and how to talk to her.

Your partner can relate to them as they are also going through or have gone through pregnancy before. Sometimes, she doesn't need answers; she only needs time to vent. Mama communities can provide her with a cozy place to do that.

Tip:

Keep the active listening tool always in use, as the mama community may be the reason for some small doubts.

EMOTIONAL SUPPORT: THE ANCHOR IN THE STORM

Dad, think of you as the trusty anchor in the storm for the ship. Your role is to keep the ship where she needs to be amid unexpected storms. You will see moments when your partner faces doubt, anxiety, fear, and sometimes happiness. You are the anchor that helps keep her grounded no matter what. Empathy and care help you be that anchor.

Dealing With the Rain of Doubts and Confusion

Things that form an umbrella against negativity:

- When she's feeling doubt and anxiety about being able to parent correctly, be reassuring.

- When she's having body image struggles and low self-esteem, show her love and reduce those concerns. Remind her you are there for her, no matter what.

- Spend quality time with her, whether a quiet evening dinner at home or an adventure outdoors.

- Surprise her with unexpected gifts to show her you always think about her. Small acts of kindness are what make the difference.

- Keep a stash of tissues. When she's mumbling some alien language and you can swear you don't have a single clue why she's crying for hours, use those tissues for a noble cause.

- When she's having mood swings, use empathy to find what may help her overcome them. During those mood swings, she may feel angry, sad, or excessively happy. Encourage her to do things that can help her overcome those feelings.

Excessive happiness can also be a concern, as people can do things they shouldn't do when they are too angry or happy.

Encourage Self-Care

It's common for our partners to stay sad for days or weeks in pregnancy. Here's a tip: She can get low, but don't let her stay that way too long. Encourage self-care and remind her to perform things that help improve the mood.

Tip:

The goal is to get her out of such moods. If she likes hanging out with some relatives or friends, invite them home. Or you can try to take her out for dinner. Whatever works is okay.

Encourage Moving That Body Around

Exercise can be a great helper when it comes to low moods. Whether it's morning sickness, hormones, or just negative thoughts, exercise is like a superhero to combat all of them. It can be tempting for your partner to avoid exercise when things get tough, but that's a slippery slope, my friend.

Not only does it affect your partner's physical health, but it also gives those negative thoughts a chance to party in her mind. And we don't want that!

So, here's the plan: Encourage your partner to take walks outdoors. The fresh air works wonders, trust me. It's like a breath of positivity that sweeps away the bad mood. Plus, her body releases these magical chemicals called endorphins when she exercises. They are like little mood boosters that can turn her frown upside down. Remember, when it comes to supporting your partner, it helps to match chemicals with chemicals.

Encourage Rest

Tiredness can make anyone cranky. When she feels her mood is deteriorating, support her in getting adequate rest. It may be challenging for her to sleep during Act 1 and somewhat in Act 3 (due to her belly), but encourage her to take naps whenever possible. While it may be difficult for her to rest fully, even a little rest can help her mind feel more comfortable and less irritated.

Pro Tip:

Lighten your partner's load by helping with household chores, cooking, and running errands.

Encourage Small Pleasures

Ever heard of someone being hangry? Don't let a lack of food lead to undesirable outbursts. The importance of a good diet can't be overemphasized, but treating her to something she likes is good if it helps with her mood. Don't guilt her over some small pleasures.

Note:

A pretty rare case is the mama having extreme negative thoughts for several weeks; it's most likely depression. Try your best; if that doesn't solve the condition, take her to a therapist.

Giving Yourself Some Slack

A super dad like you is still a dad going for the first time through the pregnancy experiences. You can try to do things perfectly, but some days can be remarkably energy-draining. Naturally, you may not always be able to maintain patience.

Just like you shouldn't beat her up over her tantrums, you should not beat yourself for some slips now and then. When you do slip, just dad-up and apologize. Then, find ways to reconcile.

I don't know about the others, but this three-act play is a team play. Moving on, we'll navigate health insurance and doctor appointments in the next chapter.

Notes

TAYLOR ANTHONY

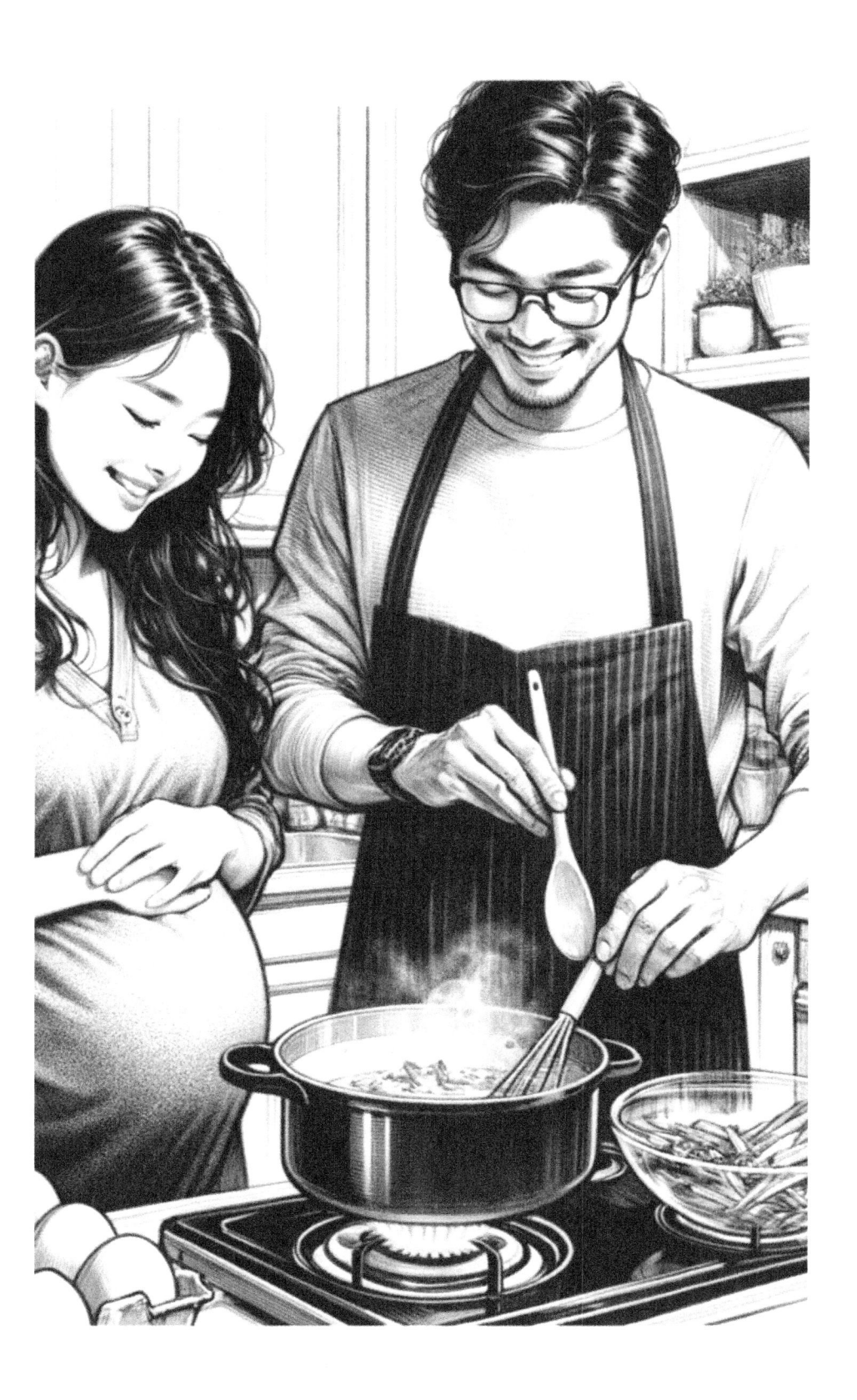

Chapter Three

The Dad, the Doc, and the Baby Bump - Tackling the Healthcare Labyrinth

"Fathering is not something perfect men do, but something that perfects the man."

— Frank Pittman

First-trimester screening may seem like a fancy TV show marathon for the first trimester, but don't be fooled, new dads! It's not about binge-watching some series. During pregnancy, you will encounter all sorts of new terms that can leave you scratching your head. But fear not! Understanding these medical terms can actually be super helpful. It will guide you on when to join your partner for appointments and even help you choose the right insurance plan. Now, I know the world of medical jargon can be a bit intimidating, but don't fret. As we have mentioned before there is an extended glossary of terms at the end of the book, that will have you sounding like you could be on staff in the prenatal department in no time.

We're here to break it down and make sense of it all!

CHOOSING THE ROUTE AHEAD

The classic route in the adventure is going with an obstetrician-gynecologist (ob-gyn).

Obstetricians focus on pregnancy, gynecologists focus on general reproductive health; hence, doctors with certifications in obstetrics *and* gynecology are called ob-gyns. Cool right? Anyways, they all belong to the professional organizational club called The American College of Obstetricians and Gynecologists (ACOG). You can check any doctor's certification for obstetrics and gynecology on ACOG's website.

Although they are the classic route, some alternative ways exist in the dadventure. A popular course is going with midwives. Now, midwives can be a great option in some situations, like if the pregnancy gets a low-risk pregnancy tag in the starting ultrasound wizardry and checkups. People with low-risk pregnancies prefer midwives because midwives are

- budget-friendly.

- all about the natural process.

- able to give longer sessions and extra tips.

Similarities Between Midwife and Ob-Gyn

Whether you go the midwife or the ob-gyn route, the pregnancy journey is pretty much the same. Both of them are like a drama with a buildup toward the end.

Both will have about 10–15 visits stretched across 8 months. One monthly visit until around week 28. Then, it will become twice like double trouble until week 36. Finally, it will be face-to-face every week. Like a normal show, there's an increase in anxiety and doctor visits at the end.

On that note, I want to mention a twist regarding midwives. Although midwives are known for those marathon-like sessions, it's a good idea to learn more about midwives as not all of them are the same. There are many types of midwives, and just like with different flavors of ice creams, you don't want to get an allergy by picking the wrong one. When selecting between midwives, first see if they

- have a good overall reputation.

- are covered by your insurance plan.

- are accredited by a reputable organization.

- have a plan B with a doctor in case a cesarean section (C-section) is needed.

Note:

The first two points also hold for the ob-gyn.

The Doctor Visits: Knowing When to Tag Along

There are many similarities between the midwife and doctor route, but I will zoom in on the ob-gyn route to simplify things. Your partner will become a close friend of the doctor during this period, and you should also add the doctor to your friend list by going with your partner to those appointments.

However, life happens, and you may not always make it due to work and other matters. No worries, though. I will share a sneak peek of what will happen on these visits. Think of it as a mini crash course that tells you what to expect during doctor visits. Like this, it will be easy to catch up if you miss anything, and you will try extra to get to the more important ones.

Higher Importance

- The first appointment is the official curtain raise of the show. It's a long session with many tests that check for infections, blood group, overall health, lifestyle issues, infection history, past travel locations, and genetic problems in the family. As I said, it's essential to be transparent with the doctor. However, human memory can be weird sometimes, and your partner may forget to mention or misarticulate some vital thing. That's where you, the eagle-eyed partner, come in. You have been living with her and know all her little habits and details. You are her trusted sidekick, but it's important to fess up about possible problems, as the health of both Mom and Baby depends on this. Doctors can suggest better solutions with all the info.

- First-trimester screening in weeks 11–14 consists of necessary tests (one being ultrasound) that can reveal whether you are dealing with a double entry like twins or a single one. The doctor may use the screening result to ask for further tests.

- Ultrasound days are the exciting part of the movie. The first ultrasound is around 10–12 weeks, and the second can be around week 18. These ultrasounds are our golden tickets to see how the little peanut is doing and how the pregnancy is going. The twins, triplets, or more come to the screen, and it's a chance to witness them. It's like seeing the baby's debut—a real-life and better version of the movies.

- Some pregnancy days are worse than others. You should be there for the particularly stressful days for the mama. That's where your support comes in. You should not miss any appointments when she's like that. One cause for worries can be the different infection checks from time to time. They help determine if any genetic defect can transfer to the child. Dangerous-sounding things like Down syndrome, gestational diabetes, and so on are checked in tests.

Sometimes, the doctor may throw out the option of optional diagnostic tests. For instance, If a test suggests increased chances of chromosomal abnormality in the baby, you may be offered diagnostic tests for definite results. They will usually inform you of the associated risk factors and then ask whether you want to push ahead. For example, some of these optional tests may increase the risk of miscarriage.

Tip:

It may be a better idea to let these go if you are going forward with the delivery, whatever the result will be—it's an unnecessary risk in that case. However, you should consult your doctor before making a decision. Also, when you go to appointments, bring snacks, tissues, and your best dad jokes. Laughter can reduce stress and make the breaks much more pleasant.

Lower Importance

Just like cliffhangers, some appointments have tests whose results you can know afterward, such as

- a glucose test anytime in weeks 24–28 to check gestational diabetes.

- a biophysical profile along with non-stress tests in the

third trimester to decide the time of delivery.

- maternal serum screening (optional) anytime in weeks 16–20 for detecting baby defect risks.

And many more. Checking blood pressure, calculating weight gain, measuring the abdomen to check the infant's growth, checking the fetal heart rate, checking hands and feet for swelling, feeling the abdomen to find the position of the fetus (later in pregnancy), urine tests and blood tests are some things that are done often on visits.

Now, here's the thing: Lower priority doesn't mean you don't need to comfort and listen to your partner's concerns. It's important to know what went on each visit, even if you missed it. Also, both lists are for low-risk pregnancies. Special cases like these raise the priority of all appointments (Mayo Clinic Staff, 2022g):

- age higher than 35

- overweight or underweight, based on BMI

- bad lifestyle choices like smoking cigarettes, drinking alcohol, and using illegal drugs

- health conditions before pregnancy, such as diabetes, autoimmune disorders, high blood pressure, cancer, and HIV

- multiple pregnancies

Guideline Regarding Doctor Visits

You may see you and your partner panicking over some test results. I hope it doesn't happen, but for example's sake, let's say a glucose test comes positive and reveals that your partner unfortunately has gestational diabetes. Or the baby's at higher risk for some genetic disease/infection.

Here's a pro tip for those occasions: Before making conclusions and overthinking things, hit the brakes and ask the doctor for clarification. Often, the situation is not what we think it is in medical diagnoses.

Why Shouldn't You Assume Things During Appointments

Let's take the case where the test result for gestational diabetes returned positive. You should ask for clarification regarding:

1. What does that mean for the pregnancy?

2. What do you and your partner need to do?

Now, gestational diabetes may seem like a scary plot twist. But this particular ailment temporarily affects pregnant women. With some caution in diet and lifestyle, it won't harm the baby and will not be carried after pregnancy (Mayo Clinic Staff, 2022d). Gestational diabetes can raise the risk of diabetes after pregnancy, but proper diet can reduce the relapse risk tremendously, the Mayo Clinic further explains.

So, whenever your partner or the doctor informs you of something worrying, first of all, calm down. Then, make your partner calm down. Finally, dig deeper with the doctor. Don't shy away from asking for clarification. Sometimes, the doctor may advise rest and relaxation. In that case, don't shy away from turning to family for help. Involve your parents, friends, and relatives if needed.

Some General Terms to Be Aware Of

Each appointment may have new medical terms you have never heard of. It may almost seem like you need to learn a new language. Asking for clarification about terms during each session is an excellent way to learn things. It's like taking baby steps toward learning a new language. This will help you get in-depth knowledge of things as they come, and you won't be overwhelmed with remembering so much medical knowledge all the time.

Remember, you are a first-time dad, and it's okay not to be a walking-talking medical dictionary. You have the doctor and, to a lesser level, the internet for help. You can try to cram everything, but half of medical knowledge can cause misconceptions and unfounded worries. There's an old joke about how a person with a fever read a medical book and thought he had all the diseases except those that occurred only in women!

With that said, it's still easy to become especially worried about the medical mumbo-jumbo at the starting checkups, so I am listing some of those terms in the glossary at the back of this book for them to become easier to digest later.

Tip 1:

Many terminologies are specific to the end of the third trimester and labor. Give yourself time to learn them so as not to overwhelm yourself. It's fine even if you learn them gradually in the second trimester. Pregnancy is a marathon, not a sprint. Also, it would be best to bookmark the glossary at the end of the book for reference throughout the pregnancy stages.

Tip 2:

It's a good idea to not dive deep into information about twins and triplets until the doctor confirms the situation. If the ultrasound reveals you are dealing with twins, triplets, or more, it's better to clarify with the doctor what they mean for the pregnancy and what you can do. Just like before, assume less and ask more. Twins come in different packages; the guidelines change depending on their type. Also, this rule can be applied generally—don't dig too deep into things that are not relevant. Mental health matters are super important, so give yourself some slack and keep things slow.

ADVOCATING FOR YOUR PARTNER: ENSURING HER NEEDS ARE MET

As a new dad, you need to become the superhero advocate for Mama's needs during pregnancy. Mama can get extra vulnerable due to physical and mental exhaustion, and your mission is to fight for her needs and ensure she receives the essential care. Let's dive into what that care includes.

Taking the Necessary Tests

This may seem a given, but timing matters for tests as well. Longer delays should be avoided, from pregnancy confirmation to follow-up appointments. For people not on health insurance, test costs can be pricey.

Health insurance is recommended, but it's extra essential if you can't afford about $19,000 for pregnancy costs (Dingel et al., 2022). That amount is the average pregnancy cost without health insurance. So, if your partner doesn't have health insurance, it's better to get that sorted.

If you have no clue, don't worry. We are going forward on this journey together, and I will give guidance on navigating the maze of health insurance later.

Emotional Anchor at Work

A part of being the emotional anchor at every step of the process is:

- going out on prenatal appointments with her and being with her when she waits for test results. It's like saying *I am with you every step of the way.*

- asking the doctor for clarification on medical terms and the future game plan. Showing you understand things helps your partner ease up as well.

- reassuring her worries regarding risk factors. It's like being the voice of reason, reminding her (and yourself) that doctors work with probabilities and not certainties.

- meeting her emotional and physical needs. This one's the game-changer. Listening and being empathetic toward her physical and emotional needs. Sometimes, it's as simple as a hug or listening to her worries.

Tests can make you and your partner go through a roller-coaster of emotions. Some may indicate a lower risk for one thing and a higher risk for another. Remember to ask for clarification from the doctor. Often, they are just probabilities and not definite things. You should be the emotional anchor and put things into perspective for you and your partner. Hey, don't end up treating small bumps like giant walls.

Meeting Her Emotional and Physical Needs

Advocating also means making her comfortable physically and emotionally; at home and in the hospital. The opportunities to do that can come in different ways:

- going to get those middle-of-the-night snack runs, foods, medications, and becoming the craving-satisfying hero.

- taking out soft pillows, giving foot massages, and making cozy blankets available are your secret weapons.

- listening to her talk about her concerns or whatever she wants. Don't forget the reassuring hugs and empathy.

However, my friend, mastering the art of listening to your partner's worries and comforting her is one piece of the puzzle. Another piece involves cross-verifying and listening to the doctor. Yep, that's right, the medical expert.

You can create a supercharged action plan by combining your partner's concerns with the doctor's input. And what does this action plan do? Well, it helps you ensure the health of both Mama and Baby. Now, part of the action plan is getting the insurance! We will dive into that below!

UNDERSTANDING HEALTH INSURANCE: SIFTING THROUGH THE PAPERWORK

Health insurance can reduce the average pregnancy cost by about two to three times (Dingel et al., 2022). It's like the superhero cape that reduces incoming damage by over 50%. The reason behind the reduction is the Affordable Care Act passed by the Obama administration.

Because of this, the registered health insurance companies can't charge extra on health insurance just because your partner is pregnant. Pregnancy is not considered a "disease," so health insurance can be applied on the health insurance marketplace whenever there's an open enrollment period—November 1 to January 15 for most states. You should check it for your state just to be sure.

Here's the game plan: If you and your partner are trying for pregnancy, or she's already pregnant, you should enroll your partner in a health insurance plan in the open enrollment period. If this period is missed, she may not be able to register for health insurance until she gives birth.

The birth of a child can fulfill the criteria of special enrollment for health insurance. However, you won't benefit much from health insurance at that point.

Breaking Down Pregnancy Costs

A lot goes into pregnancy visits: ultrasounds, glucose tests, prenatal supplements, genetic testing, infection testing, medicines, checkup fees, and other screenings. The 30 days post-pregnancy are also considered part of pregnancy costs because of the following:

- stay of 2–4 days at hospital

- administration of baby care, first tests, and so on

- visits to a pediatrician to receive newborn care and different tests

- visits to a lactation consultant within the first few weeks of delivery

Importance of Health Insurance

There are many things in pregnancy: Excitement and worries of being a first-time dad, having to juggle work and new responsibilities, and taking care of your spouse (plus unborn baby). Adding financial concerns on top of that can become a bit overwhelming. The good news is that insurance can make the average $18,000–$25,000 pregnancy costs to $2,500–$3,500 out-of-pocket costs plus $4,000–$7,000 premium.

If you are a health insurance expert, that's great, but if you are feeling a bit lost about it, don't worry. Let's break it down together.

Understanding Health Insurance

Things like *deductibles, premiums, and copays* are terms associated with health insurance.

The insurance plan becomes active when the premium is paid for the health insurance plan, say $4,800 for the year or $400 monthly.

When you buy medication or take tests, the costs are divided between you and the insurance company. Let's say the deductible is $100, and the bill comes out to be $400. Then you pay the $100, and the insurance company pays $300. This means you meet your deductible, and the insurance company pays the rest of the bill. Copays are also like deductibles. For example, let's say the bill for a doctor's visit comes out to be $100. You may need to pay $20 and the insurance company will pay the rest of the bill.

Different plans have different ratios of deductibles, premiums, and copays. Often, the health insurance plans that employers give are most cost-effective. It's worth seeing whether you or your partner qualify for them.

Other than that, Aetna, Blue Cross Blue Shield, and Cigna are three popular options for selecting health insurance plans. It's difficult to recommend one because they have different plans and coverages. It's possible that Aetna's network may not cover the hospital near you and the other two's network may cover it, and vice versa.

With that said, I think Blue Cross Blue Shield has an edge. You may find another of the two or any other reputable company that serves your region more suitable.

Tip:

Remember to check with the hospital and doctors by *calling or in-person* to find out the coverage. It's better to not rely on other confirmation sources, as they can be outdated or inaccurate.

Note for selecting a plan:

The higher you pay for premiums, the lower you pay for deductibles and copays. If the open enrollment period is around the corner, and you find out that Mom is pregnant, it can be a smart option to get a high-deductible health plan (commonly known as HDHP) if the pregnancy is lower risk. Higher-risk pregnancies should consider the higher premium plans. If you are unsure about the riskiness of the pregnancy, it may be better to select a plan with a moderate premium.

For Very Low-Income Families

You may qualify for Medicaid or a similar insurance program if the family's financial status is low-income. You should check your eligibility for these plans when considering health insurance plans.

PREPPING FOR THE DELIVERY ROOM: WHAT TO EXPECT

The delivery room is like the final boss room, so there's bound to be tension. But you should do your best to remain calm. You and your partner's comfort becomes very important there. You will want to maximize your comfort by

- wearing comfortable clothes
- reassuring yourself
- pacing around nervously (pun intended!)

You may see more dads in comfy T-shirts, sweatpants, and sneakers. You want to be relaxed and focused on you and your partner's comfort instead of minding other things (e.g., dress and food). To do this, you should bring a functional backpack.

Preparing for the Delivery Room: Dad-Style

The Dad Bag

This bag should contain snacks, a phone charger, a change of clothes, a set of clothes for the baby, and a good book like this one. The hospital only serves meals for the mom, so most snacks are yours. The baby will come out eventually, but the wait can be painful. You may watch the clock cross hours to become days. If you are staying the night, also bring a jacket and long pants (even in Summer), as the hospital thermostat may be set to cold.

Documenting the Moment

Part of following dad-style to the T is capturing the first moments with your child. You should take some photos and videos to remember this incredible experience in the future. Try to use tech only for this purpose and put it down whenever possible. That's the tech etiquette at the birth location.

Finishing Touches on Dad-Style

Dad-style involves comfy clothing, but it's more than that. It's about handling the emotional whirlwind: excitement, nervousness, tension, and overwhelming love. Relish them and show mental resilience.

You can show mental resilience by being ready for things beforehand. For example, you will have higher mental resilience if you visit the delivery place a few times before to familiarize yourself with the environment. Even small actions like securing the baby's car seat show mental resilience and preparedness. Being ready will help you become relaxed, and things will feel more natural.

As I said, practicing makes this three-act play perfect. There will be unexpected things, but part of dad-style is being prepared as much as possible to adapt to the situation better.

The goal is to advocate for your spouse by following medical advice and supporting her choices. It's one of the best times to unleash your dad jokes and spread humor. It can help you and her relax. If she likes conversation, engage in it to distract her mind from pain. Reassure her as much as needed!

With that, we will explore together how we can navigate morning sickness, the other big challenge of the first trimester, in the next chapter.

Notes

PREGNANCY GUIDE FOR FIRST-TIME DADS

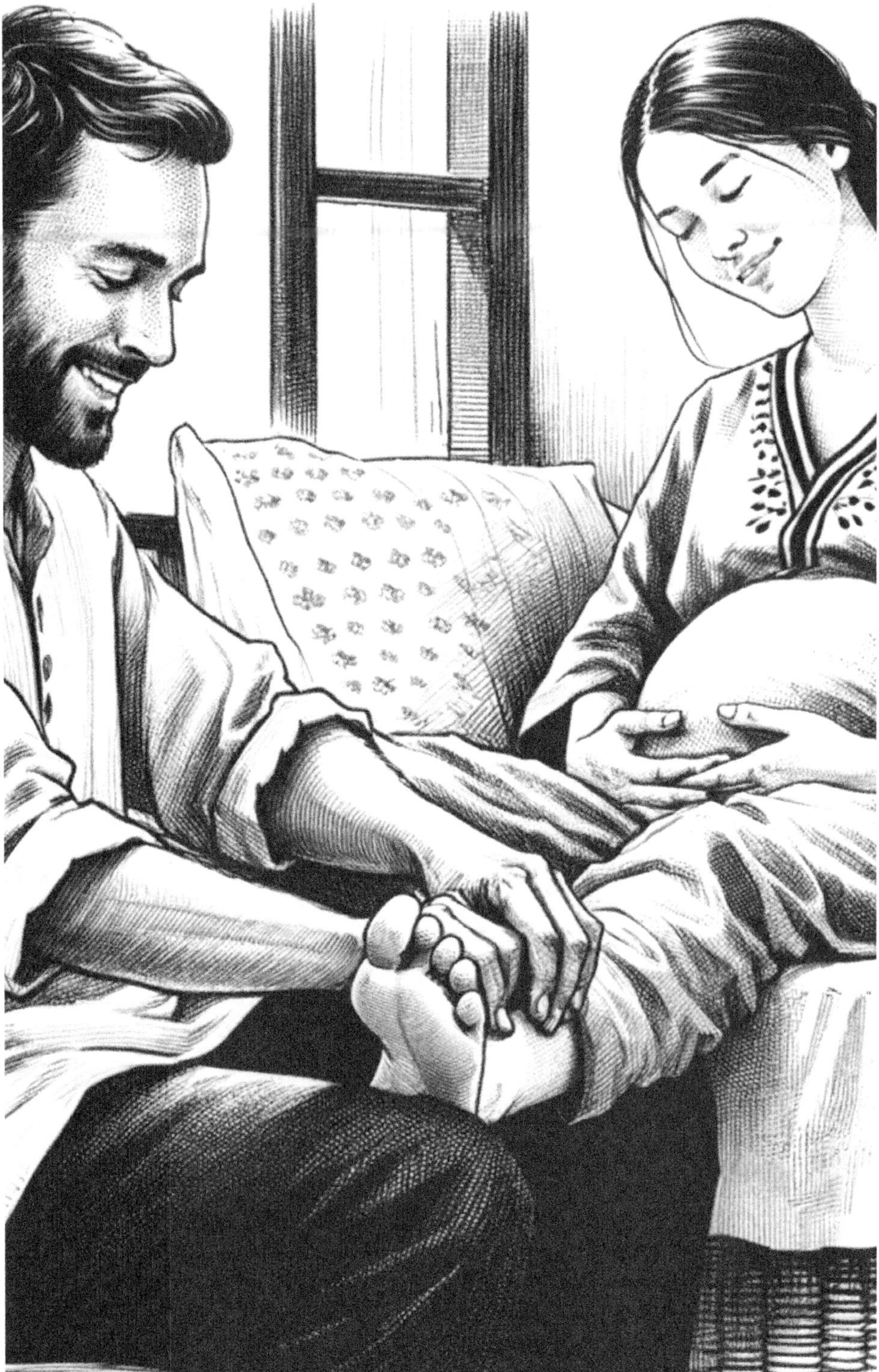

Chapter Four

Navigating Nausea - Making Queasy Easy for First-Time Dads

"Morning sickness: because 'all-day, everyday sickness' wouldn't sound as catchy."

- Unknown

Alright, fellas, let us dive into another side of the world of pregnancy. Chapter 1 spilled the beans on interesting changes, like the magical breast swelling and the never-ending bathroom trips. Don't worry, though. Your partner can still handle them!

Things get a bit trickier when morning sickness and mood swings crash the party. These two troublemakers can mess up the well-being of both Mom and Dad. We have already tackled mood swings, so it is time to conquer morning sickness. Buckle up. It is time to get into the trench.

UNDERSTANDING MORNING SICKNESS: THE WHAT, WHEN AND WHY

It's no secret that pregnancy can turn even the most robust stomachs upside down. Now, if morning sickness only happened in the morning, it wouldn't be such a headache.

To grasp the concept of morning sickness, picture motion sickness. It's like having something lodged in your throat, ready to appear at any moment. This alone brings constant physical and mental discomfort, but a few more companions come along for the ride, just like a gang sticking together. They are:

- hunger pangs
- reflux
- exhaustion

Even though the package sounds like complete trouble, there is a bright side to it as well.

Morning Sickness: A Positive Pregnancy Indicator

Morning sickness in pregnancy can be a bit like a quirky recipe. It may seem like a strange mix of ingredients, but the result is worth it, as I mentioned in Chapter 1. The early pregnancy nausea serves as a sign of a lower miscarriage risk. Wondering how it's connected?

Well, when the pregnancy-specific hormones rise significantly, it's common for women to experience nausea and vomiting. Almost 4 out of 5 mothers feel some level of nausea during this time—some more, some less (Bustos et al., 2016).

Morning Sickness: When Does It Strike?

Some good news! Morning sickness is not a permanent condition throughout pregnancy. It typically starts around week 6 for mothers and peaks between weeks 8 and 12.

It then subsides between weeks 12 and 16 and rarely returns. Important to note is that even when morning sickness is at its strongest, not all mothers experience daily nausea and vomiting. If a mother is vomiting frequently, like 3–4 times a day, contacting the doctor without delay is a good idea.

Note:

A minority of mothers may experience morning sickness throughout pregnancy. This is more common in high-risk pregnancies with twins or triplets.

Morning Sickness: The Real Fangs of the Beast

Vomiting and nausea during pregnancy lead to a lack of bodily fluids and exhaustion. The more severe the symptoms of morning sickness, the more alarming the fluid loss. If your partner doesn't try to consume extra fluids, dehydration quickly becomes an issue. Encourage her consumption of fluids by giving her soups, shakes, or smoothies—whatever is easier for her.

Tip:

While water and other fluids are good, if they are difficult to consume or make her nauseous, foods with water, like melons, are a great option.

UNRAVELING THE SCIENCE BEHIND MORNING SICKNESS

Understanding the science behind pregnancy can help dads navigate morning sickness with more ease. We know that increased levels of pregnancy hormones like estrogen, progesterone, and hCG play a role. Now, many food and lifestyle choices can make the symptoms milder, but they can't make the symptoms go away completely.

Why Can't Medications Work Their Magic?

That's because of two main reasons:

- We don't want to disturb the natural hormonal changes.

- Research on morning sickness is not that detailed currently.

So, don't have your partner take any strong over-the-counter medicine like pain meds, sleep aids, and so on without consulting the doctor. The doctor will determine, considering the symptoms, whether they should prescribe anti-nausea medications or not.

Things That Make Morning Sickness Worse

While factors like the rise of hormones are beyond control, some things are controllable. For example, morning sickness worsens when Mom is

- stressed.
- overtired and sleep-deprived.
- in warm weather.
- on an empty stomach.
- stuffed with food.
- low on blood sugar or water.
- frequently traveling.

Warm temperature can be like a trusty sidekick to morning sickness, causing loss of fluids and exhaustion.

Also, thanks to the hormone pair estrogen and progesterone, your partner's body suddenly became a food processing factory on overdrive. These hormones relax digestive tract muscles, causing inefficient digestion and giving your partner metabolism changes and hunger pangs.

Now, morning sickness can affect any pregnant woman, but it can be more severe in high-risk pregnancies, such as those with multiple pregnancies due to the higher hormone levels in the mother. It's all about the hormones!

HANDY AND PRACTICAL FIXES FOR A CHALLENGING PROBLEM

Although we can't do much about the hormone rise, there are several ways to mitigate the symptoms of morning sickness. They mainly involve food, mindset, and lifestyle improvements, with a sprinkle of prenatal vitamins.

Healthy Food: The Number-One Guideline Always

Good food and lifestyle remain the lifeline throughout the play. That includes staying away from alcohol, tobacco, marijuana, and so on. Foods that will be helpful follow almost the same guidelines: high in protein, low in grease and spice, low in fats, and easy to digest.

If all else is failing during morning sickness, consider a combination of the following foods, as they can be easier to digest:

- bananas
- rice
- soups
- applesauce
- boiled potatoes
- lean chicken
- yogurt
- boiled veggies
- toast

Tip 1:

One good combo is bananas, rice, applesauce, and toast, short form BRAT.

Tip 2:

Salt aids digestion, so eating some salty foods can be really helpful.

Snack Attack: Conquering the Day With Small Bites

It turns out that both a full and an empty stomach can lead to unexpected bouts of nausea. Imagine this: Your partner just devoured a hearty meal, only to find herself hunched over the toilet, regretting the waste of food and energy.

One time, I'd prepared a sumptuous meal of roasted chicken with a side of carrots. The moment she laid eyes on the plate, she shot off faster than a bolt of lightning. I was left alone, listening to the echoes of retching sounds from the bathroom. The chicken and carrots were demoted to being my lunch for the next three days.

To avoid this unfortunate scenario, consider smaller snacks throughout the day. Eating smaller snacks guarantees that some food gets digested during the day, as the fast metabolism helps digest quickly.

Additionally, it ensures that your partner's stomach is never left empty. Trust me, an empty stomach can be a recipe for a truly unpleasant vomit experience, which is both painful and utterly exhausting. So, in summary, embracing smaller meals will provide Mom with a steady stream of energy and help minimize the not-so-fun side effects.

Tip:

Ensure six or more small meals instead of three larger ones.

The Mighty Ginger at the Rescue

Ginger deserves its spotlight because it's like a savior in reducing the severity of morning sickness. Ginger comes in capsules, candies, tea, and other forms, making it easy to consume. Trust me, taking liquids with ginger in them can work wonders most of the time!

Dive Into the World of Endless Hydration

A healthy lifestyle without fluids is like a sandwich without filling. You have probably heard the generic "drink more water" a million times, but useful things are meant to be repeated. The health benefits of consuming water and other fluids are many in morning sickness, where losing liquids is very easy.

Find out which temperature water your partner is comfortable with and keep that ready to roll. Often, slightly icy cold liquid (and sucking ice cubes) can be extra easy on the throat. Room-temperature liquid is usually preferable, but it's much better to have some liquid than no liquid!

Minding Those Scents

It's no hidden secret that nausea can be worsened by smell. So, it's best to put away and wash out whatever smell causes her nausea to take a nosedive. The tricky part is that, like allergies, some of these triggers vary from mom to mom. Here are a few common culprits:

- spices from food while it's being cooked or after it's cooked

- strong perfumes that attack the nose

- smoke from a cigarette or cooked food

- smell of mold in a damp environment like the washroom

- strong pet odors

- smell of gasoline

On that note, not all smells are created equal. While some smells can be unpleasant, others can be refreshing and help with nausea. For example, the refreshing scent of peppermint and citrus fruits like lemons and oranges can usually give relief. Furthermore, eating sour candies and lemon drinks is worth a try, too!

Adopting a Pro-Health Lifestyle

Other than eating healthy food, avoiding nauseating smells, and drinking a lot of fluids, healthy lifestyle guidelines also help reduce the effects of morning sickness. They include stuff like not:

- lying down right after eating.

- eating too much or too quickly.

- ignoring brushing teeth.

- taking excessive stress.

- depriving the body of rest.

Some vomit material can get stuck in teeth and cause bad breath, which can reduce the appetite and become the precursor to further nausea. That's why brushing your teeth multiple times daily can be helpful for your partner. Also, not brushing right after eating can be a good idea.

For most of these points, you can give her timely reminders in case she forgets. To help her get the rest, you should help in the house whenever she's tired or sleepy.

Managing the Use of Prenatal Vitamins

Sometimes, your partner may feel queasy after taking those routine prenatal vitamins. A simple solution? Offer her a snack to have with the vitamins. Another trick is taking the vitamins right before bed or at a time when she often feels less nauseous.

But hey, we have got more options! You can consult the doctor about the use of chewable or gummy versions of the vitamins.

Still, if all else fails with some pesky prenatal vitamins, don't just skip out on those nutrients. Ask your healthcare provider about alternative ways to get the iron and vitamins your partner needs during pregnancy.

Also, safety first! Don't take any new supplements before checking with the doctor.

Out-Of-The-Box Methods

Acupuncture and massages can help the body relax, which is useful but not completely necessary. However, some hypnosis can be significant. Not the kind where they say, "You are feeling sleepy," but the one that helps alleviate concerns about morning sickness. Stress and fears related to morning sickness can be physically and mentally draining, disrupting sleep and potentially worsening the effects of morning sickness. If you can reassure her with constant positive talk, that's the best hypnosis we can hope for.

EMOTIONAL SUPPORT DURING MORNING SICKNESS

Remember I mentioned tagging along with your partner in stressful appointments? Appointments around morning sickness days can be exhausting, so providing emotional and physical support is crucial during these appointments. Morning sickness usually peaks by week 12 and becomes rare after, so it's only 1–2 appointments.

Be prepared to talk about how often she has nausea, how often she vomits, whether she can keep fluids down, what's her diet, and whether she tried any home remedies. Sometimes, just having someone explain things on your behalf is an excellent source of emotional support.

Empathy: Feeling Her Discomfort

Empathy is key again, guys. As I mentioned, it doesn't come naturally to us what she's feeling because of the hormone imbalance. What she's feeling is not just motion sickness; it's motion sickness on steroids.

To bridge the gap, empathy is crucial. You may have seen ramps made for physically disabled people before. The idea behind them is not to neglect their needs and to ease their problems. I am not saying treat her like some disabled patient fellas; instead, show care by putting in some effort.

For example, one practical way to deal with motion sickness is for your partner to eat smaller snacks throughout the day. It would help if you used empathy to consider all the situations where you can assist her with that information. One way to help is to always carry a bag of snacks when you are out with your partner. Or you can make and store healthy meals to help her get a balanced diet. Hey, you can let her take a rest from household chores when you feel she's sleep-deprived or tired. It's really about feeling her situation and listening to her concerns.

This all shows that you care about her needs and plan accordingly. The handy tricks I mentioned show their full effect when used side by side with empathy.

Emotional Support in Your Absence

Since you won't always be available at home due to work and other commitments, consider asking a family member or friend to assist your partner. This will provide her with emotional support, someone to talk to, and someone to help with her food and other needs.

WHEN TO SEEK MEDICAL HELP

Nausea and vomiting can keep anyone wondering when to call the doctor. It's normal for pregnancy nausea to be somewhat bad. Here are a few standard things:

- feeling nauseous for some time each day
- vomiting once or twice in the day

Shedding Some Pounds Is Possible

Even if a woman loses some pounds in the first trimester instead of gaining the recommended 2–4 lb, that's still not something to be panicky about (Lindberg, 2020). The lost weight can be made up in Acts 2 and 3, so the baby isn't harmed.

What if Your Partner Doesn't Experience Morning Sickness?

Hey, dads-to-be, here's a little scoop on morning sickness: As mentioned, around 20% of moms experience little to no effects (Bustos et al., 2016). If your partner hasn't experienced morning sickness by week 12, high chances are it won't come.

While its absence doesn't affect the baby's health after birth, it may raise concerns about whether hormones are rising correctly. Make sure to mention these details to the doctor so they always have the information to guide the pregnancy.

But What's Considered Abnormal?

Experiencing frequent rounds of vomiting during morning sickness can lead to a loss of some pounds for Mom. However, even this weight loss should be within healthy limits. Although severe cases of morning sickness are very rare, you should know the symptoms just in case. The signs to look out for include (Cleveland Clinic, 2023a)

- nausea lasting several hours each day
- losing around 10 lb or more
- vomiting four or more times per day
- producing no urine or only a little urine that's a dark color

- inability to keep any liquid down

- feeling dizzy or faint when trying to stand up

- having a high heart rate

- vomiting liquid that's brown like it has blood in it

Special Tip for Appointments in Morning Sickness

Keeping notes on the daily routine and diet, including food and supplements, is a good idea during pregnancy. Hypothetically, let's say that mom suddenly experiences severe morning sickness symptoms. Notes can help determine the exact cause of the symptoms.

It may be the case that it happened naturally, or it may be the case that some smell, food, or supplement was the trigger. Severe symptoms don't necessarily occur because of a natural cause. The detailed notes also help the doctor suggest other supplements, foods, and lifestyle habits.

Notes also have the advantage that they help remember things and give answers to the doctor. For example, notes can help you respond if the doctor asks:

- Do symptoms occur at certain times of the day or randomly?

- Do you notice specific triggers for nausea or vomiting?

- Does anything make her feel better?

Tip:

The notes are handy not just in morning sickness but also throughout the pregnancy.

Hey folks, although morning sickness is a sign of a healthy pregnancy, it can drain a lot of energy if we let it. Smells can trigger nausea, so it's best to be mindful of them. Healthy food, plenty of water, small meals, good rest, and a healthy lifestyle should be your partner's friends to manage morning sickness.

With that, we are done with the main problems of the first trimester. The second trimester is like a calm and peaceful cruise. Throughout the book, I have recommended things to buy—you can buy those things in the second trimester. The third trimester can be a bit tricky, so we will dive into the third trimester in the next chapter. Get ready to witness the mind-boggling and mind-numbing changes of the third trimester!

Notes

PREGNANCY GUIDE FOR FIRST-TIME DADS

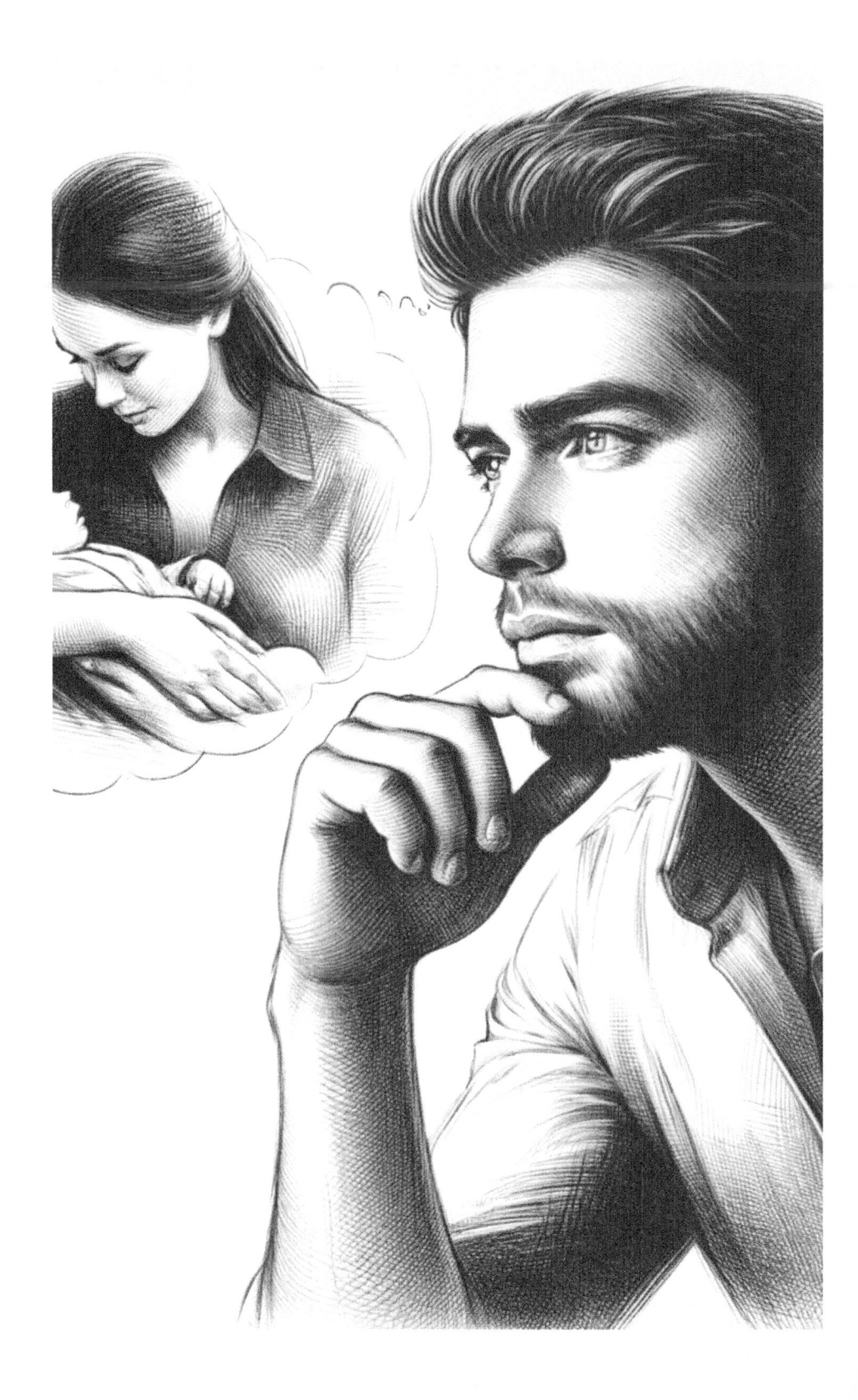

Chapter Five

The Home Stretch - When She Waddles, You Hustle

"The most important four words for a successful marriage: 'I'll do the dishes."
— Unknown

Let us take a moment to review what we have so far. We looked at mood swings and morning sickness, the power couple of the first trimester. We also peeked at what happens in the second and third trimesters. And now, brace yourself, because the third trimester is like the boss battle of pregnancy challenges.

THE CONTRAST BETWEEN CHALLENGES OF THE FIRST AND THIRD TRIMESTER

The challenges of the first trimester for new dads are that mom is still getting used to all the pregnancy changes, and everything feels new. Many medical terminology and worries are circulating in her head (and yours) as she goes through the initial appointments and tests.

She's also experiencing morning sickness and mood swings for the first time, which can prove to be a roller-coaster emotionally and physically... and by roller-coaster, I mean the kind that makes you scream, laugh, and question your life choices all at once.

Then, the second trimester comes to the rescue, giving both of you a much-needed break. It's the easy-going part of pregnancy where you both can focus on buying things for your little one. And hey, the baby equipment you need to buy is discussed in Chapter 11.

Coming back after the break, the third trimester starts. Once again, it starts to hit both of you that you will be Mom and Dad soon. This wait may feel long, but don't worry. Before you know it, you will hold the baby in your hands. Also, this wait is not the only bump for you and your partner.

The problems of the third trimester are like multiple ants working together. They each play their small part in making your partner go through physical and emotional turmoil. They include physical problems like body pains, insomnia, exhaustion, heartburn, and constipation, and emotional ones like the fear of birthing pain and coping with the worries of being a good mother. The physical and emotional aspects are both important, and I have got you covered. Ready? Let's go.

THE LATE PREGNANCY BLUES: UNDERSTANDING YOUR PARTNER'S DISCOMFORTS

The first mystery in the third trimester is when the baby will make their entry. The baby also wants out of that tiny room, and they appeal their case for early release by constantly making movements.

It's natural to eagerly await the next stage, but here's the catch: Navigating the treacherous waters of pregnancy in the third trimester is like trying to find your way out of a corn maze! Multiple signs seem to say that the birth is about to happen. These signs can raise expectations, only to dash them repeatedly, especially during the last few weeks.

However, we still need to look at these signs and how to navigate the physical changes. By understanding and dealing with these changes, you can help reduce the agony your partner has to endure until the big day.

Physical Changes: Embracing the Symphony of Backaches and Full-Body Pain

The saying "no pain, no gain" also holds in pregnancy. The baby's size and position can often cause discomfort to your partner. Many of the physical changes are the body's way to ensure a smoother pregnancy. Pain can occur in seemingly every part of your partner's body during this time—from her back to her hips to her stomach. There are so many places that may feel like a wrecking ball has hit them. It's like a full-body workout, but without the six-pack abs to show for it!

However, sometimes, physical pains go beyond preparing the body for pregnancy; they indicate preterm labor (the term for delivery before week 37). They are indicators and not a done deal, which sets the stage for the cycle of expectation and wait. In summary, the signs are (Mayo Clinic Staff, 2022a)

- moderate abdominal cramps like menstrual period with/without diarrhea

- one Braxton-Hicks contraction every 10–15 minutes for a total of 4–6 times in an hour

- change in the type or amount of vaginal discharge, such as watery, mucus-like, or bloody

- flu-like symptoms such as nausea, vomiting, or diarrhea, like not being able to tolerate liquids for more than 8 hours

- constant ache in lower back that doesn't go away even after about an hour of rest

- pelvic pressure as if the baby is pushing down hard

- come and go lower backache that doesn't go away by changing position

Note:

A special case is the baby going into ninja mode after week 28. Doctors typically recommend you tell them if the baby makes less than 10 movements (e.g., kicks, twists, or turns) in any 2-hour period. It's not preterm labor, but a sign that the baby's growth needs to be checked.

Braxton-Hicks Contractions

It can feel like someone is squeezing and twisting muscles, causing discomfort or a dull ache in the lower abdomen. These contractions are there to make the birthing process easier. They are like the trial runs before the final run, increasing in frequency as birth comes closer. Although it's normal for pregnancy to reach 37 weeks and above, 1 in 10 pregnancies go through labor before that time in the third trimester (WebMD Editorial Contributors, 2022). This means one important thing. If around week 36, 4 weeks before the due date the doctor gave, your partner feels 4–6 contractions within an hour (or other labor signs), it's time to run for the doctor. It's a strong indicator of preterm labor.

Mind you, they are not intense tear-jerky pains but more like discomforting pains. If the pain becomes severe, it may be a sign of some infection for which you still need to run to the doctor.

Vaginal Pain

These pains may make mom anxious, so it's better to give her extra attention when she's having vaginal pains. It's like a puzzle that keeps both of you guessing—is it a false alarm or something more? But hey, don't panic too much, and stay on the lookout for the following signs so that you can contact the doctor ASAP:

- piercing pain in the vagina
- vaginal bleeding
- pink or brown discharge
- pelvic pressure as if the baby is pushing down hard

Backaches and Hip Pain

Hormones continue to increase to make for a healthy delivery. Remember, I mentioned that hormones could loosen the body? They loosen the connective tissues between bones, enhancing pelvis flexibility and making the boss baby entry easy. But hey, as they say, all good things come with pain. These changes can be tough on her back and can easily cause discomfort. The back pain brings along its trusty sidekick, hip pain, as the body posture starts to resemble a wobbly penguin due to the back pain. Signs of preterm labor in this case are:

- intense back pain

- dull lower backache that stays even after 1 hour of taking resting positions

- feeling pressure radiating toward the thighs

- come-and-go lower backache that doesn't go away by changing position

Frequent Trips to the Bathroom

Did you know that as your baby grows, they can put some serious pressure on your partner's bladder? And let me tell you; it's not just a physical change in this case. It can be a cause for some emotional damage, too!

The extra pressure can make her leak, even with the tiniest actions like laughing, coughing, sneezing, bending, or picking something up. So, if you forgot to stock up on panty liners during the second trimester, now's the time to make a mad dash to the shop! And hey, don't worry. Some trickling is likely just pee. It only becomes a sign of preterm labor *when the discharge amount is unusual, like spilling a large glass of water. This extra water can come out at once in a burst or slowly.*

Tip:

Some of the preterm labor signs have room to be misinterpreted as being due to other reasons. For example, gas pains can also cause pain in the lower abdomen. If you have a basis to think the symptoms match preterm labor signs, you should contact the doctor immediately. Is there a possibility it may turn out to be a false sign? Definitely, but it's best to be on the safe side, as delaying in case of real labor can cause complications.

Pains That May Require Medical Attention

Other than the pains that make you go through the cycle of expectation and disappointment, more physical pains pop up during the third trimester. Here is one that can have you reaching for the phone to call your doctor.

Leg Cramping and Restless Legs

Muscle pain in the leg can happen because of a nutrient imbalance—too much phosphorus and too little calcium (Nall, 2018). This may be due to the overconsumption of meat and the underconsumption of dairy and fish.

Restless legs seem like their mischievous sister, but they are not. It's that constant urge to move one or both legs, and it can be because of iron or folic acid deficiency, Nall (2018) explains. Now, they both are important in pregnancy, so contact the doctor if your partner shows spontaneous activities like:

- restlessness

- a strong urge to move one or both legs

- nighttime leg twitching

Pains That Are Just Chilling at the Party

Some problems don't require urgent medical attention. They are like attempting to change a diaper in the dark. Challenging, but ultimately, we navigate through them. They are described below.

Severe Lack of Sleep

Imagine sleeping with an outstretched belly and multiple body pains. If you imagined that, great. Back to reality, these things naturally lead to difficulty in sleeping. This lack of sleep, in turn, causes exhaustion. This, in turn... okay, no more.

But let's not forget the joy of snoring! Yes, snoring can also happen as the baby's size can pressure those poor breathing muscles.

Note:

Don't take medications for insomnia. If the doctor advises some medicine, take only that in the recommended amount.

Tingling in Buttocks, Thighs, and Lower Back

Being a new dad comes with some unexpected perks—like discovering all the nerves in the body! On that note, let's not forget about the sciatic nerve, which gets extra attention thanks to the enlarged uterus.

It might give your partner a tingling, numbness, or even a little pain in her lower back, buttocks, and thighs. This can happen on one or both sides of her body.

Spider Veins, Varicose Veins, and Hemorrhoids

Do you like spiders? You may need to because your partner may now look like a spider woman. Tiny red-purplish veins can appear on her face, neck, and arms due to increased blood flow. And hey, if swollen veins appear on her legs, they are called varicose veins. But wait, there's more! If they appear in the rectal area, they change their name and become... (drumroll)... hemorrhoids!

Tip:

Foods with fiber can help a lot, like brown rice and oatmeal. For hemorrhoids, hazel pads, sitting in a warm water tub, and some ice can relieve the pain. For varicose veins or swelling in the legs, your partner should reduce the time spent standing and putting pressure on the legs.

Stretch marks: Stretch marks can also appear around the stomach, breasts, buttocks, and thighs. They may seem like distant relatives of spider veins, but they are caused by the skin not being elastic enough (Marcin, 2023). Don't worry, though! Just ask your partner to gain weight gradually and apply lotion. These marks will naturally fade away (mostly) after the little one arrives. It's like a magic trick but without the wand!

Shortness of Breath

Being a new dad is quite the experience. It's like seeing a human's body suddenly becoming a loose puzzle.

Mom will get pressure on her breathing muscles and will have a baby bag that will seem to have taken up permanent residence in her stomach. No wonder you will find her huffing and puffing even with the slightest physical activity. You might even see your partner returning from the second floor, thinking she just conquered a marathon!

But fear not, dear dad! Helping her with exercises to improve posture can give her lungs some much-needed room to expand and catch their breath.

Heartburn: Not the Emotional One

Hormones wreaking havoc can cause heartburn. The valve between the stomach and esophagus (the esophagus tube connects the stomach to the mouth) decides to take a vacation and relax, allowing stomach acid to rise—we call that heartburn.

And guess what? Heartburn is a bit of a food critic!

So, if your partner is experiencing heartburn, it's time to investigate if she's missing out on some of the goodies from the healthy menu and healthy eating habits we mentioned for the first trimester. Particularly, avoiding fried foods, citrus fruits, chocolate, and spicy foods is a must. Also, eating small meals helps, just like in morning sickness.

Heartburn in the second trimester: Heartburn can also happen in the second trimester, and adopting the same diet can help.

EMOTIONAL SUPPORT IN THE THIRD TRIMESTER

The third trimester can demand a lot more rest from your partner, giving her mind time to reflect on good and bad thoughts.

Other than physical pains, anxiety about birth pain can become persistent. *How much will it hurt? How long? Can I cope?* Dealing with your partner's emotional turmoil is all about reassuring her and keeping her busy. And hey, if she starts worrying too much, hold her hand and remind her that you will be there to hold her hand during labor… and maybe even squeeze it a little too tight if she starts getting on your nerves! But remember not to go overboard.

Tickling Time: Keeping Your Partner Busy …. and Happy!

The mom community she joined before can be the reassuring agent she needs. It's like when you are not the only one with a fever in class—it suddenly feels a little better. Plus, having someone to share concerns and excitement with is an emotional remedy.

The journal I recommended can also keep her busy noting down and planning things. Give her lots of good material to think about:

- If breastfeeding, how will she do that—a nursing bra or a breast pump?
- Who should they ask to help around with the baby?
- What should be the limit of visitors?
- Who will be the pediatrician for the baby?
- What are her birthing preferences (birthing plan)?
- Are things prepared in the home for the baby?

- What are her plans for 40 days after delivery?

- How can she cherish these last weeks of pregnancy?

- How can she embarrass the little one when they become an adult?

- Has she mastered the art of diaper changing and putting babies to sleep?

These work along with exercise, short walks, napping, cooking, and frequent showers. The final finishing touches to this are you spending date nights with her. This can be going on long night walks, watching movies together, or having a great home-cooked dinner at home.

Tip:

After all that, if busying her is still needed, a hobby like trying out new recipes, reading books, or learning a new skill (e.g., language) is an option.

PRACTICAL WAYS TO HELP WITH PHYSICAL PAINS: FROM MASSAGES TO OPENING YOUR WALLET

The list of pains may have raised some concern, but here's the good news: There are plenty of ways to lessen their effects. Knowing them equips you with the secret weapons you need in your arsenal. But before that, let's get to know the enemies. Insomnia, leg pain, backaches, and hip pains are four significant dark horses to deal with. Though, don't worry!

With a dash of humor, a dose of preventive know-how, and the addition of empathy, you will conquer them like a true diaper-changing superhero.

Tickling the Sleepless: The Misadventures of Insomnia

The human body has an incredible power to self-recover when it gets proper rest. As a dad, one of the best ways you can help is by assisting with rest. A good sleep routine is to sleep and wake up at fixed times. It is even better if your partner can sleep early at 9–10 p.m.!

But as always, there's a catch: pregnancy pains can throw a wrench in this plan anytime. It's like those pregnancy pains have a wicked sense of humor, you know? They are like mischievous little gremlins, poking and prodding just when she's about to enter dreamland.

And let's not forget about the alarm clock in the middle of the night. But it's not your typical beeping sound, oh no. It's the sound of her bladder, demanding to be emptied for the umpteenth time.

But wait, there's more! Just when she manages to settle back into bed, your little bundle of joy may decide it's time for a dance party. Who needs sleep when they can have a private concert in their belly, right?

So, if you find her wide awake at 3 a.m., contemplating the mysteries of the universe and wondering why she ever thought sleep was important, remember that you are seeing something natural.

Still, some guidelines can aid in getting better sleep:

- Remind her to drink lots of fluid 2–4 hours before bed and little to no fluids within the 2 hours before bedtime.

- Massage her feet a little before bedtime and aid or ask her to stretch her legs before bedtime.

- Remove foods that contribute to leg cramps from the shopping list, especially removing carbonated (like Coke or 7 Up) and caffeinated drinks (like tea or coffee) for yourself at home can make it easier for her to stop taking them (Nall, 2018).

- Encourage her to take left-side (better for baby) or right-side leaning sleeping postures.

- Remind her to take a bath in warm water right before coming to bed.

Tip:

When she's lying on the sides, ensure a soft pillow underneath the belly as support. If she has heartburn, try putting pillows under her upper body.

Don't Force Sleep

Still, sleep can sometimes seem out of reach. When she really can't sleep, forcing it is unlikely to work. Instead, busy her with a relaxing activity in bed, as that can prepare the body for sleep. You can keep her entertained with hilarious dad jokes while in bed! Laughter is the best medicine, even for sleepless nights! Some of the other things you should try:

- giving her a book to read
- talking to her for some time
- asking her to do something that you know relaxes her

Tip:

Sleep quality guidelines obviously should be followed. Like being in a cold, quiet, and dark room—hey, you can even use curtains and earplugs to transform your bedroom into a sensory deprivation chamber. Also, no use of the mobile screen 1 hour before bed. Trust me, having her scroll through dad jokes won't help her sleep. And let's not forget, no focus-intensive activities like work activities and gatherings 1–2 hours before bed.

Note:

No sleep insomnia medications before consulting the doctor. Those medicines can be quite addictive.

Backaches and Hip Pains: The Harassing Villains

The best way to deal with backaches and hip pains is to mind the posture. As a new dad, you should avoid asking your partner to do things that risk disturbing her body posture. For example:

- lifting heavy objects
- bending down at the waist
- wearing high-heeled shoes

Some things that make her posture better are:

- when walking, using low-heeled, but not flat, shoes
- if squatting, bending knees as well
- when sitting, using chairs with good back support (and maybe a cushion) and a stool as a footrest
- when sleeping on sides, putting a cushion between the legs

- when standing, standing straight and not drooping

- before sleeping, getting a massage

- when exercising, doing exercises for back muscles—exercises that you consulted with the doctor beforehand

- when awake, wearing a maternity support belt

Leg Cramps: When Muscles Decide to Dance Without Permission

Leg pains are a significant hurdle to getting good sleep. Reducing them can help fight against insomnia. Some things that reduce leg cramps:

- eating calcium-rich foods (e.g., milk or cheese) (Marnach, 2023)

- avoiding straining legs by activities like crossing legs, wearing tight clothes, wearing hard or high-heeled shoes, and so on

- stretching legs and calf muscles with light exercises

- getting some good old massages and applying a hot water bottle to the sore area

Note:

It's always best to avoid sleeping on the back and stomach. The first may disturb blood flow, and the second can put pressure on the spine.

Hemorrhoids

A simple strategy to prevent hemorrhoids and to prevent their worsening is:

- not sitting on hard surfaces for long periods
- avoiding putting strain when emptying bowels
- taking smaller meals and avoiding constipation
- avoiding tight underwear or pants

Tip:

Taking more fiber and fluids helps with constipation.

Perky Transformations: Breast Changes

Breasts get bigger to produce milk for the baby. Bluish veins can appear on them, nipples will darken, and a thick yellow fluid can start to leak—some perfectly normal changes. This can be tackled by having

- supportive or cotton bras

- bras of different sizes that match breast size and don't irritate nipples

- cotton handkerchiefs in each bra to absorb leaking fluid

Tip:

Buy nursing or maternity bras, as they provide amazing support in these aspects and are usable after pregnancy.

Note:

Remind her to clean her breasts using warm water without extra products like soap. Anything more may cause irritation or itching.

Vaginal Discharge: A Comedy of Unexpected Surprises!

Mostly the same as with breasts: avoid tight pants, wear cotton underwear, and clean the area with warm water. Soap can also be beneficial if it doesn't irritate.

Note:

Using pressurized water to clean inside the vagina is a no-no. It can cause unnecessary complications.

FINAL THOUGHTS

And that concludes the all-rounder information overload you need to stay on track in the third trimester. Your role is to share reminders with your spouse and do what you can. This can include buying things, giving her massages, setting a date day, and being on the lookout with her for signs of preterm labor and medical problems. This removes the burden from just being on your partner, and you both divide the responsibilities as a team—although her share will still be heavier overall.

Notes

TAYLOR ANTHONY

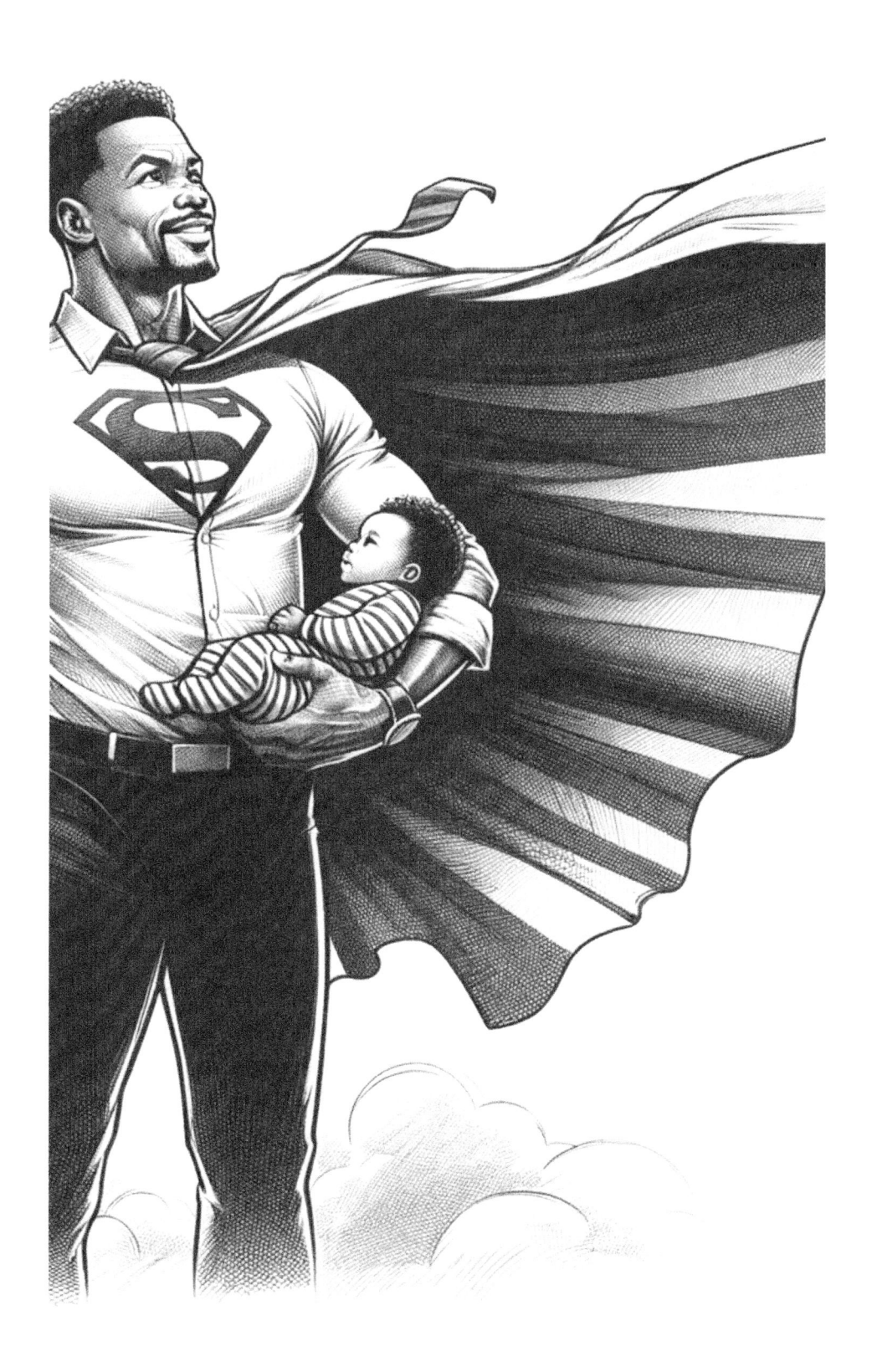

Dads Helping Dads

Hey There, Fellow Dad!

You know, being a dad for the first time is a lot like trying to put together a puzzle without the picture on the box. It's exciting, baffling, and, let's face it, a little scary! That's why I wrote "Pregnancy Guide For First-Time Dads." It's your friendly guide through the maze of pregnancy and early fatherhood.

I've been where you are, wondering why babies cry at 3 AM and how to make sure my partner feels supported and loved. It's a journey filled with highs, lows, and lots of learning. In this book, I'm sharing everything I've learned – the good, the not-so-good, and the "I wish someone had told me this sooner" stuff.

Now, here's where I need a tiny favor from you.

Can You Help A New Dad Out?

There's a new dad out there, just like you were, feeling a bit lost and looking for guidance. You can help him! How? By simply sharing your thoughts on this book.

Your mission, should you choose to accept it:

Please leave a review for "Pregnancy Guide For First-Time Dads."

It's super easy and won't take more than a minute. Your review could be a lifesaver for a dad in need. You'll be helping another dad navigate this exciting time, and who knows, your advice might just make his day (or night) a little easier!

Here's How To Do It:

Step 1: Grab your phone and scan the QR code on the next page.

Step 2: Share your honest thoughts on the book.

Step 3: Pat yourself on the back for being awesome!

That's it! You've just made a huge difference in another dad's life.

Welcome to the Dad Club!

TAYLOR ANTHONY

If you're the kind of person who loves to lend a hand, you're definitely my kind of guy. You're now an honorary member of the coolest club around – the Dad Club!

I can't wait for you to dive into the next chapters. There are so many neat tricks and heartwarming stories waiting for you.

A big thank you from me, Taylor Anthony, and dads everywhere. Your support means the world.

PS: Remember, sharing is caring! If you think this book could help another dad, why not spread the love? Pass it along and make another dad's journey a bit brighter!

Chapter Six

Embrace the Chaos - A Newbie's Guide to Unpredictable Joys of Fatherhood

"Never is a man more of a man than when he is the father of a newborn."
                           - Matthew McConaughey

We all know that first-time moms experience a wild mixture of emotions during pregnancy and after. But dads are not immune to these changes either. I mean, even taking a big exam or going to your first job interview can be stressful, right? Well, guess what? First-time fatherhood is no exception!

We go from being our average selves to someone with a new set of responsibilities. It can be like having to navigate through a dimly lit maze, which can make any dad-to-be a little anxious. But fear not, because I have your back, just like always!

UNMASKING THE FEAR: COMMON WORRIES FOR FIRST-TIME DADS

Dad Fears, the greatest hits album of fatherhood anxiety, can be divided into six categories.

1. Am I going to be a good dad?

2. Will we be okay financially?

3. Is the baby going to be ok?

4. My social life is going to take a dive.

5. I won't have sleep or personal time.

6. Will mom be alright?

If you are feeling a confused mix of these, don't panic; you are not alone! I again welcome you to the wild and wacky world of new dadhood! Now, let's unpack these fears like a pro.

AM I GOING TO BE A GOOD DAD

The fears of being a good dad span over a lot of things. From wondering if you can master the art of unconditional love to figuring out how to wade the waters of parenting, it's a wild ride. We are here to tackle these fears, one at a time!

Fear 1: "Will I Do Everything Right?"

Any father can care for their child. Even cavemen raised their kids, and they were pretty rugged—not to mention they didn't have any parenting books like you do. So, if you don't know how to change diapers right now, no worries! You'll be able to learn it.

But hey, will you always make the best decisions? Well, that's a reasonable misunderstanding. Sometimes, those decisions make for great photo opportunities, like when you end up bathing the baby in the sink.

Now, getting more knowledge and practice will definitely help you become a better dad, but you will have to quit that perfectionist mindset in some things. It's okay to put the baby in front of cartoons for an hour to save your sanity. Nothing to feel bad about there. And hey, if you feed him something sweet just to watch his adorable reaction or to get him to stop crying, again, nothing to feel wrong about. We've all been there. And let's not forget the moment you will be late picking up the baby from grandma's (or relative's) house because you *really* need a nap. Trust me, *nothing to feel worried about.*

Fear 2: "Will I Be a Good Father?"

Fathers usually fall into two categories: Those who want to parent just like their own dad or those who want to do the complete opposite.

It's like they are divided between wanting to be a mini version of their old man or breaking the cycle. And to be honest, it can be pretty overwhelming. Thoughts like, *How am I supposed to do this?* or, *My dad never did it for me, how can I do it?* creep in. But hey, don't keep it all bottled up inside. Talk about it. Share your worries and problems out loud.

What are the things you don't want your kid to inherit from you that you got from your dad? Or what are the obstacles that are stopping you from being the superhero dad you always want to be?

Remember, we humans are great problem-solvers. By identifying and working on those challenges, you will definitely get closer to becoming the father you want to be. Maybe you won't be the perfect role model you envisioned, but you will become the role model your little one needs. It's just like what Norman Vincent Peale (n.d.), a writer with fantastic work on positive thinking, said, "Shoot for the moon. Even if you miss, you will land among the stars."

Fear 3: "I Wouldn't Be Able to Love Unconditionally or Give Them Enough Attention"

Here's the thing: You haven't had that baby in the house yet. You don't know that the baby is in a kind of similar SOS situation. They may look at you first like, *Who the hell are you?* Often, they may only recognize Mom. There hasn't been enough time to build a baby-to-dad bond. After their arrival, it may take months, but both of you won't be able to resist giving in to the love.

Side Note: There will be a whole chapter on work–life balance, so don't worry about insufficient time.

Fear 4: "They Will See Me as Inadequate and Flawed"

Hey, the reality is that your kids are not going to be born with a superpower vision to scan all your flaws. You can always hide those few things you don't want anyone else to figure out.

And the best part: Kids have this unique ability to ignore flaws. They are like teenagers with their superhero obsession.

They can brush off anything strange as cool and anything wrong as *it doesn't matter*. Dad, you're the superhero for your baby, and it will stay that way if you do their upbringing correctly. Kids ignore flaws and instead see the time and care you put into them. Your love and hard work leave a lasting impression on their little minds.

Fear 5: "Can I Teach My Kid the Things They Need to Grow Into a Healthy Adult in Today's World?"

Let me tell you, being a great dad is indeed a challenging task. It's like trying to grow a baby plant—you need knowledge, time, effort, and the right conditions.

The fact of the matter is that no matter how hard you try, there will always be some things that are out of your control. If you have a daughter, she might grow up obsessed with the Kardashians. If you have a son, he might be all about video games or sports, no matter his background. Or maybe your child will positively exceed your expectations.

Your job is to do what *you can do*, and to be the best dad *you can be*—a dad who teaches them morals and how to be good humans. They may not be the exact copy you imagined, but with a positive upbringing, they will be ready to take on the world!

Fear 6: "I Don't Want to Deal With Those Diapers"

As a new dad, you may find yourself questioning whether you can be a great father if you hate the thought of dealing with those stinky diapers or a baby who could unleash vomit at any moment. But hey, who can blame you? It's like facing the horrors of the universe! But fear not, my friend.

With time, you will adapt to things, just like any other challenge. Maybe you will create a designated baby playroom, or perhaps you will have a separate wardrobe just for carrying the baby. Or maybe you will simply embrace the art of carrying them around like a pro. Trust me, by the end of the day, you will be an expert at handling those explosive situations!

Fear 7: "I Don't Know What to Do"

How can I help Mom? What can I do for the baby? These are good questions to start with, but not ones to stop at. Confusion is cleared by seeking answers, and you can quickly become informed. You can ask Mom straight away what she needs help with. Easy-peasy right?

Also, you read a book on pregnancy, and you got terrific clarity (by the way, now is an excellent time to help other dads by giving a great book review). Just like that, you can get additional books to bridge any knowledge gap. Books are a close friend, so keep them that way.

And remember the dad community you joined before? It would be best if you stayed connected with them to stay in the circle. The more you know, the more confident you become. And here's the thing: Sometimes, you don't need information. You only need a simple conversation to ease your fears.

WILL WE BE OKAY FINANCIALLY?

Fear 1: "I Fear Not Being Able to Provide for the Family When There Are Kids"

Don't worry. You are not alone in thinking that your bank account is going to file for bankruptcy. Parenthood comes with its costs, but there are ways to reduce them.

Now, just get an idea of what you must spend on, and you can create a budget that won't make your wallet cry. Yes, just like how you normally make a budget (minus the impulse buys). Consider the following things for a budget:

- baby essentials (mentioned in Chapter 11)
- healthcare costs (discussed in Chapter 3)
- cost of a nanny if both of you are working
- loss of income in case of parental leave
- your insurance plan
- Dad-Joke Fund (discussed later in this chapter)
- household expenses and groceries
- transportation costs

Once you have a budget, there are plenty of ways to save money. Joining Facebook Marketplace or scouting for second-hand toys and prams on eBay can save a ton of cash. Remember, being a first-time dad means mastering the art of budgeting. Forget about fancy gadgets; your baby will be just as happy with a cardboard box and a set of keys. Trust me, they will find joy in the simplest things.

Having a game plan in front of you can relieve severe stress and improve mental clarity. Plus, it will help you avoid spending frivolously like a contestant who's just won the lottery on a game show. So, embrace your inner financial wizard, because you have got this!

Pro Tip:

Not every baby tech gadget is necessary. Always remember: You have the power of negotiation! Do your homework before splurging on anything. You don't want to end up with a fancy-looking thing that collects dust in the corner while your wallet weeps.

Fear 2: "My Quality of Life Will Decrease"

Your concerns are valid. But here's the thing: once that little bundle of joy arrives, it's like someone turned up the saturation and added a whole bunch of vibrant colors to your world. Suddenly, there's more joy, happiness, and anticipation in your life than you ever thought possible. There will be a sense of fulfillment and achievement with every little milestone.

From the first smile to the first steps, each moment will be a victory for you and your baby. The monotonality of life will decrease, and you will feel alive like never before, as your attention shifts to this tiny human who has stolen your heart.

But here's the best part: Becoming a dad doesn't just make you a parent; it also makes you a better person. You will become more patient, compassionate, and in tune with the world around you. Suddenly, it's not just about working for yourself anymore. You are now on a mission to prepare a new life that will positively impact the world. It's hard for life to get more fulfilling than this.

Fear 3: "I Will Have to Pay for My Child's Wedding and Education"

Oh no, the dreaded fear of paying for their wedding and education!

Here's a lighthearted perspective to put your mind at ease: Remember, you have plenty of time to plan and save for these milestones. Your child's wedding and education are years away, so there's no need to panic just yet. Take a deep breath and listen.

As far as education after high school is concerned, remember, there are various options available. Scholarships, grants, and financial aid can help lighten the burden. Plus, your child might be a genius and earn a full ride to university. Or they may earn a good portion of fees through a part-time job or small business. Who knows? The possibilities are endless!

What about their wedding? Picture this: your child, all grown up, standing at the altar, ready to say "I do." As a loving dad, you might find yourself reaching for your wallet, only to discover that your child has already found their perfect match, who happens to be a billionaire! Problem solved, right? Well, maybe not. But like I said, you have plenty of time to save and there are many possibilities. Your child will also be in a position to pay for their own wedding when they are an adult.

But wait, there's more for the saving mind! Embrace the power of humor and start a Dad-Joke Fund. Every time you crack a cheesy dad joke, put a dollar in the jar. Not only will it lighten the mood, but it will also serve as a small contribution toward those future expenses. This dad-joke fund doesn't only have to be added on with jokes. You can also set aside some percentage (5%–10%) of your salary for this fund and invest it in stock indexes like S&P 500.

So, dear new dad, let go of that fear and embrace the journey ahead with a smile. With a little creativity, negotiation skills, dad jokes, and a knack for saving, you will navigate the financial challenges of childcare like a pro.

IS THE BABY GOING TO BE OKAY?

Fear 1: "Something Will Be Wrong With the Baby"

It's just like a quote by Debasish Mridha (n.d.), an American author: "Fear comes from the lack of knowledge and a state of ignorance. The best remedy for fear is to gain knowledge." Remember the stat about the chances of miscarriage after the first trimester? Yes, close to zero chances.

Now, throughout pregnancy, moms undergo all sorts of tests and treatments to ensure their and their babies' health. It's like taking a sneak peek into the future. Are there some unknowns? Of course, because life is full of unknowns. But you should chat with your healthcare provider and get some stats whenever something is worrying you about medical conditions.

Trust me, once you have the facts, you will realize that the annoying kids running in the neighborhood are not some rare phenomenon. Instead, they are the norm. So, get those stats from your caregiver when you are worried because they are the kryptonite for those pesky fears.

Fear 2: "We May End Up Hurting the Baby"

Babies may look fragile, like a touch may cause blood leakage, but they are actually quite tough. Firstly, they can handle common colds without any significant issues, and they won't suddenly drop dead without warning.

Even if something happens, like falling from the bed, some kisses and pats can calm the situation. Let's imagine a scenario where the situation gets a bit more serious, like a little blood involved. Some bad fall, for instance. In such cases, the essential kit mentioned later in Chapter 11 can help. Not to mention, pediatricians are there to handle such situations. Remember, falls are pretty common, yet countless couples have successfully raised healthy babies—you both can easily do it too!

MY SOCIAL LIFE IS GOING TO TAKE A DIVE

Fear 1: "There Will Be No Social Life and Hanging Out Anymore"

That's a little silly fear. Children are actually quite portable, and the chances are that your buddies with or without babies aren't going to just vanish. Like rebooting your device, your life system will be up and running soon. You will have something resembling a social life within the first 2 months of the baby's birth.

The math is easy. The baby is outnumbered: two of you and one of them. So, one of you can go chill when the other one is on the battlefield.

But let's be honest: socializing and late-night adventures will likely not be the same again. The mere thought of handling a crying baby at 3 p.m. and 3 a.m. leaves us with 2 options: either embrace moderation or face the consequences!

Note:

Okay, if you have twins or triplets, it won't be two against one, but the same is true: One holds the fort when the other leaves.

Fear 2: "Life With My Wife Will Not Be the Same"

That's true… because your bond will improve. Having a child builds stronger bonds in couples in some hilarious ways. Picture this: You and your partner stumbling through the house at 3 a.m., trying to soothe a crying baby. It's like a modified version of *Survivor*, where the prize is a more robust relationship! From diaper blowouts to toddler tantrums in the supermarket, finding humor in the madness will bring you and your partner closer together.

You and your partner will develop an unspoken language of eyebrow raises, secret hand signals, and perfectly timed "shh" sounds.

It's similar to a comedy act, except the audience is a tiny human who finds your antics boring. And let's not forget the ultimate aphrodisiac: Baby giggles. Trust me, your relationship will be hotter than ever!

Sure, there will be some other changes, like dad having to practice abstinence from sex beginning around the birthing period to 4 weeks after birth. Or trying to talk to Mom, but seeing she's a little exhausted. Or seeing a lot of boobs, but knowing they are not for you. Don't worry, though. Focus on being the best sidekick, and you will have things back in no time at all!

I WON'T HAVE SLEEP OR PERSONAL TIME

Fear 1: "I Will Never Sleep Again"

You will. It's the most difficult at the start, for which you both can have a secret sleep strategy. It can be one of you handling a few nights per week or month and the other tackling the rest.

Or you can tag-team, like one sleeping through the first half of the night and the other on the second half. Additionally, you can call in veteran soldiers, codenamed Grandpa and Grandma, as reinforcements to help for a few days. Your relatives can also take turns being sleep-deprived some days. It's a tried-and-tested method that has worked for many dads. Trust me, it will also work for you.

Fear 2: "I Won't Have Time for Myself"

Let me tell you something: You are already doing a great job by trying to learn to be a dad. But hey, even superheroes need some downtime to recharge those batteries. It's natural and, dare I say, necessary. You will want to have a personal space to escape and truly call yours.

It can be a small room, an attic, or a small corner in the garage. It's where you can indulge in some *me time* daily or weekly and disconnect from the chaos of dad life. Your mental health is more vital than ever, and you will often need a little relaxation time to get back into the game.

Now, I know what you are thinking. Will you have to say goodbye to your beloved beer stash or bid farewell to those epic gaming sessions? Well, maybe not. There are still ways to make things work, my friend. Sit down together and have a heart-to-heart about the top things that matter most to both of you. Then, take turns! That way, both of you can enjoy your passions and hobbies.

Being a dad doesn't mean giving up everything you love. It's about finding that perfect balance between being there for your little one and caring for yourself.

Note:

My personal opinion is not to consume alcohol if you can, but plenty of dads can still make it work when they do it moderately.

IS MOM GOING TO BE OKAY?

Fear 1: "Will Mom Be Okay During Delivery?"

Whenever any fear like this is troubling you, go to the healthcare provider and ask them for the stats. The fatality chance from delivery to 42 days after it is 0.0003% in the US (Hoyert, 2023). And that includes households where the mother had previous complications or poor economic backgrounds. So, it's like worrying about lightning striking in the middle of a sunny day. Technically possible? Yes. Is this paranoia? Absolutely.

Fear 2: "What About Postpartum Baby Blues? Will She Be Able to Cope Emotionally?"

Facing emotional upheavals after pregnancy is not too uncommon of a thing. The new responsibilities can affect the mother's mind, and when she thinks she has it all figured out, those sneaky pregnancy hormones decide it's time for a vacation!

We've got a term for these emotional ups and downs: baby blues. They are like a temporary storm cloud hovering over the mother in the first 2 weeks after birth. However, sometimes, those clouds can overstay and develop into postpartum depression. The good news is that it's treatable. The next chapter will dive into what you need to navigate those stormy clouds.

THIS TOO WILL PASS

Pregnancy's 1st year can feel like it's dragging on forever. You will be running on fumes and wondering why your baby doesn't understand your desperate SOS signals for sleep. But hey, think about how quickly the past few years flew by. The 1st year of parenthood is full of events with its ups and downs, but trust me, it will fly by too.

No matter how tough it gets, after the initial months and the sleepless nights, when you see your baby lying on your chest and looking at you, you will feel all you did was more than worth it. The joy and satisfaction of bonding with your little one and witnessing their growth will make you feel like a lucky dad. So, on tough days, remember that this too will pass and will become a cherished memory. With those fears out of the way, we will continue navigating postpartum depression in the next chapter, as I promised.

Notes

TAYLOR ANTHONY

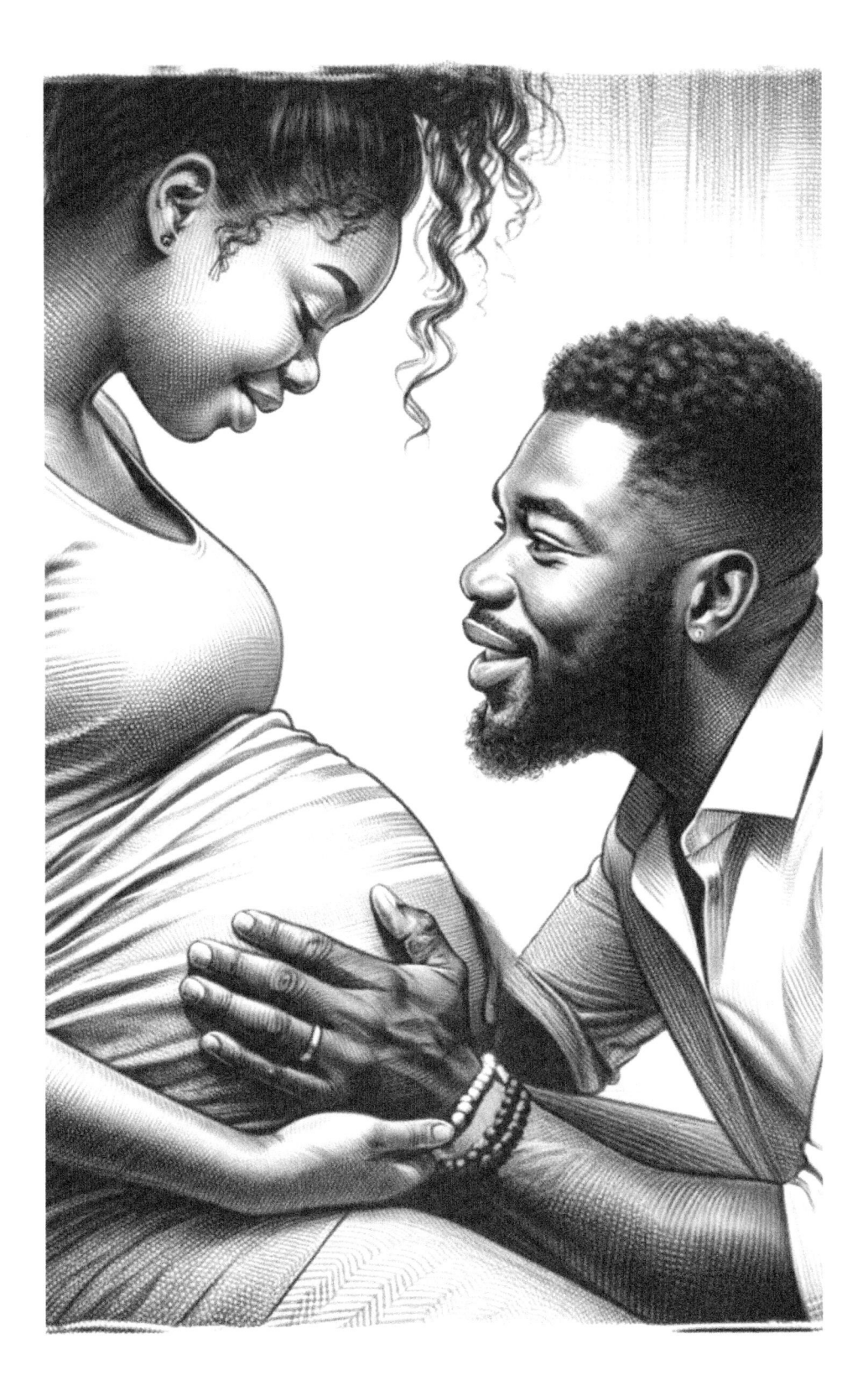

Chapter Seven

Keep Calm and Daddy On - Surviving the Emotional Rapids of the Postpartum Period

"Tough times never last, but tough people do."
- Robert H. Schuller

Whew, we've gone through a lot! We've covered how you can help your partner with the physical pains throughout the pregnancy and be there for her emotionally. But hold on tight because there's one more battle on the way: post-pregnancy depression (also called postpartum depression).

You see, about 1 out of 8 moms experience postpartum depression, and an overload of worries and problems contribute a lot to it (Office on Women's Health in the Office of the Assistant Secretary for Health, 2023). The winning formula I mentioned works wonders here: giving her the emotional support she needs, keeping her busy with activities she enjoys, and helping her resolve any concerns.

By doing so, you significantly reduce the already-low chances of depression creeping in. And hey, if she doesn't have a history of depression, those chances are even lower!

But on the off chance postpartum depression does make an appearance, remember that it's treatable! Now, we must first know how to spot the problem before we can go toward the treatment. To truly understand postpartum depression, we need to start with the after-pregnancy baby blues.

THE POST-PREGNANCY BLUES: UNDERSTANDING WHAT THEY LOOK LIKE

Put yourself in your partner's shoes for a second. Imagine you are the new mom who just had a baby—there's a lot of congratulations and applause! But hold on, there's a problem. Instead of basking in the glory, you find yourself shedding tears over diaper overflows, snapping at anyone who dares cross your path (including your poor spouse), and daydreaming about disappearing for a while without a care in the world—no breastfeeding, no worries.

My friend, these are the classic symptoms of the baby blues. It's not your partner's fault for feeling this way—about 4 out of 5 moms go through it (March of Dimes, n.d.-b). So, what's the treatment plan? Well, here's the good news: You don't need a treatment plan. It's like the after-shocks of an earthquake. These baby blues usually exit by themselves within a week or two, max. So hang in there, new dad!

Baby Blues: Hormones, Stress, Worries, and Relationships… Oh Boy, It's Like a Drama

The beginning of the post-pregnancy period is when Mom and Dad try to figure out how to fit this whole parenting thing into the routine. They face a fuel shortage; there's just not enough sleep to recharge those exhausted batteries. And those hormones? Well, they are taking a vacation after seeing a job well done. I mean, just the hormone estrogen alone can mess with mood regulation. So, these things combine to make for some interesting scenery, like seeing your partner

- feeling like crying over small triggers
- having trouble thinking clearly
- being especially irritable
- missing parts of her old life, like friend hangouts
- having anxiety about the baby's health and safety
- experiencing insomnia or restlessness even though

exhausted

Since Mom can run out of gas, it's no wonder she can feel a bit unattached to the baby. I mean, who has the energy to care about anything when they are completely drained? This results in the mom state I asked you to imagine before. But here's the good news: Moms can adapt within a few days to 1 to 2 weeks, which helps them escape the baby blues. So, hang in there and remember that a nap is the best medicine (and some laughter, too)!

Note:

Baby blues may appear 2 to 3 or more days after birth.

Make Your Way to Happiness: Things That Help

- **Sleep, and more sleep:** When the baby sleeps, she should get some z's. There's a pile of laundry? Can you give it to someone else? No one there (not even a neighbor)? Forget about it until it grows into an unignorable tower. That's because good sleep works wonders and makes things smoother.

- **Send an SOS:** When grandma or grandpa offers help, seize the opportunity and put them to work. Trust me, it's a win–win! You can assign them tasks like cooking meals, running errands, or changing diapers. It lightens your load, and it will give them a chance to bond with the little one. So, go ahead and give your partner and yourself a well-deserved break!

- **Staying fit and getting fresh air:** Mom should be rocking a fabulous body thanks to her diet and exercise routine. Encourage her to keep it up because it will keep her energized and ready to take on the baby world. And don't forget the boost a stroll in the fresh air can give her mind.

- **Talking to someone:** Picture your partner as a soda can, her emotions bubbling like fizz. You can avoid her becoming a fizzy bomb if she's engaging in daily chats with family, friends, or fellow moms who get her and won't give her the side-eye. It's like she has a support group of understanding nods, without the added burps.

- **Being preoccupied:** Rest is the key to survival, but we must keep things in check. The hormones are uncontrollable, and we don't want to give them an opportunity to steer the mind. That's why Mom should become preoccupied whenever her mind starts wandering. Hey, being preoccupied doesn't have to be all about being a 24/7 servant to a tiny human. Starting with some lovely hobby she used to do before the baby's arrival should keep her sane, give her some much-needed rest, and prevent any potential resentment from creeping in.

- **Staying connected:** Hey, new dads, squeeze in quality time with your partner consistently. Remember those date nights you used to have? Well, maybe you can't go all out like before, but you know, 20–30 minutes of fun daily or a few hours on the weekend is an excellent way to start. It's like a mini-vacation from diaper duty!

BABY BLUES AND BEYOND: THE PROGRESSION TO SEVERE STAGE–POSTPARTUM DEPRESSION

You have been doing everything to keep both your partner's and your mental health intact. The good news is that the chances of experiencing any long-lasting mental health issues are as low as finding a parking spot right in front of the grocery store on a busy Saturday! But hey, life is full of surprises, right? So, let's talk about the difference between postpartum baby blues and postpartum depression, shall we? They are

- intensity of symptoms
- total duration

You know, having worries is part of life, and some concerns now and then are likely not something to be worried about. But, suppose you see baby blues like crying, irritability, insomnia, and trouble thinking clearly, lasting longer than 2 weeks. In that case, it may be some degree of postpartum depression.

Regarding intensity, baby blues can be more like feeling a little out of sorts here and there but still being able to go with the daily routine. On the other hand, postpartum depression can be persistent and affect daily functioning.

But then again, it's not like the baby is handing out "Mama is depressed" stickers. And you won't find a neon sign flashing "depressed" above someone's head, either. Mom might just be exhausted from a long week or a sleepless night. The same goes for irritability; it's not always a sign of depression. It could just be a case of "I haven't had my coffee yet" syndrome. Now, extreme stuff like suicidal thoughts or trying to harm the baby? Yeah, that's depression, but they are not your everyday occurrences. That's why we need some ways to catch depression.

Catching Postpartum Depression Red-Handed

Now, here's a popular way to catch depression: through questionnaires! Yep, you heard me right. Just have her answer these fancy questionnaires designed to diagnose depression, and then you can tally up the score like you are keeping track of points in a game. Think of it like a mental treasure hunt.

Note:

I have given PHQ-9, a famous questionnaire for catching depression, at the end of this chapter.

The Importance of Relationships

When you have a robust family system with frequent visitors, they can be the first to spot baby blues taking a toll on the new mom. From diagnosing the symptoms to aiding in the cure, these family superheroes are here to save the day. With their timely help tackling household chores and having good chats with the new mom, they can prevent those baby blues from turning into full-blown depression.

And if things have unfortunately reached the depression stage, they can put things back on track. So, don't hesitate to call family reinforcements to help save the day.

Ways to Help: Natural Recovery Methods

Here are two reliable methods to battle depression.

Crazy Brain Tricks: Cognitive Behavioral Therapy

Cognitive behavioral therapy (CBT) may sound like a spell from Hogwarts, but it's just a way to help your partner identify those tricky thinking patterns. You see, exhaustion mixed with hormones like estrogen can mess with her thought process, leading to wild beliefs and distorted perceptions. And they can be challenging to separate from her normal thinking. CBT is your secret weapon to help your partner untangle those thoughts.

It's a proven and effective way where the goal is to lead the other person using digging questions. It's like playing detective, but instead of solving crimes, you'll be solving the mysteries of the mind.

Some of the targeted negative patterns in this are:

- guilt
- inadequacy
- self-doubt

Seeing What That Looks Like

You ask a question: Why are you feeling down? The response may be that *I am a failure because I can't handle everything.* At that point, take a step back and examine this together. Does being a superhuman who can handle everything all the time sound realistic? Well, it seems like an unrealistic expectation to me.

After coming to that conclusion together, it's time to find an alternative thinking pattern. Like telling her that instead of beating herself up, how about embracing the fact that it's okay to ask the awesome dad or relatives for help? The icing on the cake would be to tell her that she's doing her best, and that everyone makes mistakes, even the awesome dad!

This is what CBT is all about—asking questions and correcting misconceptions and beliefs. It's similar to a mental makeover, where we challenge and replace those unrealistic thoughts with more positive ones.

Tip:

Using CBT doesn't mean you have to *turn into a detective,* interrogating your wife for hours on end. Think of it as having regular conversations where you play the role of a supportive partner. You are trying to figure out what's bothering her to help her break free from that negative cycle. Plenty of resources are out there to help you master the art of asking the right questions. But if you are still scratching your head after trying to learn them, you can ask your healthcare provider to point you to a therapist.

Interpersonal Therapy

Have you ever heard that chatting is the best remedy? Well, it turns out that talking to friends and family can strengthen relationships and make you feel better.

Interpersonal therapy (IPT) is like social networking therapy. Remember that mom community we mentioned earlier? It's not just a bunch of moms sharing tips. It's a social network where moms can develop realistic expectations instead of putting unnecessary pressure on themselves. And if you and your partner have some relatives or friends living nearby, they can be even more helpful than online connections. They can lend a hand in so many ways!

Having social networks to hang out with means less time spent alone with negative thoughts. So, why not have her plan meetups and fun activities with friends? It's a great way to stay productive and keep those bad feelings and depression away.

Also, don't forget about each other. You two have the most important connection. Set aside some quality time for just the two of you. Try to recreate those date nights you used to have during pregnancy. It's a great way to keep the spark alive in many ways!

EMBARK ON A JOURNEY WITH YOUR HEALTHCARE PROVIDER

Who needs a healthcare provider's approval when you and your partner suspect she's dealing with depression? If you both feel like you are running out of options or need an extra helping hand, it's time to consider seeking outside help. Your partner can have a heart-to-heart with the healthcare provider and develop an action plan.

Two heads can be better than one, especially when it comes to tackling the challenges of parenthood.

Ups, Downs, and Side-Splits of Antidepressants

Here's a little tip: If your partner starts taking antidepressants because the healthcare provider suggested it, she shouldn't just quit them one day because she feels like it (March of Dimes, n.d.-a).

These little pills can be a bit weird, and stopping them suddenly can cause withdrawal symptoms. Only when the healthcare provider and Mom have both decided it's time to say goodbye to the meds, will the provider help her gradually reduce the dosage—like a slow-motion exit in a blockbuster movie.

Tip 1:

Antidepressants can take time to take effect, like 6–8 weeks. It's a good idea to confirm with the doctor how long your partner needs to wait to see the effects. You can ask the doctor to change the medicine if the effects don't show.

Tip 2:

Antidepressants are playing with the mind, and the mind is a complex thing. Keep your eyes open and watch your partner closely in the weeks she's taking antidepressants—to catch if something feels amiss.

POSTPARTUM DEPRESSION: DO DADS ALSO GET THE BABY BLUES?

Hey, new dads, guess what? It's normal for you to have moments of anxiety and worry. We have gone through Mama's baby blues, but guess what? Dads can have their version of postpartum depression, too. So, here's the deal: Take care of your mental health. It's like putting on your superhero cape to avoid getting overwhelmed and burnt out.

CBT, IPT, and Some Dad Time

Alright, listen up, dads! Remember those tips I mentioned earlier? They work for moms and dads alike. But let's give them a dad-tailored twist, shall we?

Firstly, set aside some time daily or weekly to analyze your negative thinking patterns. It can be 20 minutes before bed or 20 minutes in the morning. It's a time when you go through your mind without distractions. On that note, connecting with other dads, whether in person or online, can help you set realistic expectations. It's like pruning away those unrealistic ideas and misconceptions. Trust me, it works wonders.

Secondly, remember you are not alone in this crazy journey. Maintain those social connections with other parents, friends, and extended family. They are a vital support net, ready to help in many ways. The most important help is that you can count on them for their physical presence when you need it the most.

Finally, don't forget about the dad-only time. Carve out a little space each day or week to disconnect from everything. It's like hitting the reset button and giving yourself a breather. I mentioned a bunch of ideas in Chapters 6, 8, and 9 on how you can make time for hanging out with your buddies and taking care of yourself. Society gives less importance to the needs of the father's side, so you have to be the one to advocate for yourself.

And guess what? If you follow these tips, you will probably never need to turn to antidepressants. They are like the last resort, so let's steer clear if possible.

The Changing Role of Fathers

The role of a father has gone through unstoppable changes in recent decades. Society now expects dads to be more than just breadwinners. We are supposed to be mentally prepared for everything, emotionally and physically present for Mom and Baby 24/7, and master the art of raising kids while ignoring our emotional struggles. Unfortunately, society doesn't care about the fact that we can feel unprepared for all of the changes life throws at us. Talk about a tough gig! But fear not, Dad!

You don't have to please everyone. In the next chapter, we will navigate society's expectations together so that you can find your own incredible dad path. Let's rock the dad life with a smile and a healthy dose of humor!

PHQ-9 Questionnaire

The table on the next page shows the PRIME-MD diagnostic 9-question Patient Health Questionnaire (PHQ-9) (Kroenke et al., 2001):

PHQ-9 scores of 5, 10, 15, and 20 represent minimal, moderate, moderately severe, and severe depression, respectively.

If you checked off any problems, how *difficult* have those problems made it for you to do your work, take care of things at home, or get along with other people?

Patient Health Questionnaire - Depression (PHQ-9)

Instructions:

Over the last 2 weeks, how often have you been bothered by any of the following problems?

	Not at all	Several days	More than half the days	Nearly every day
Litle interest or pleasure in doing things	0	1	2	3
Feeling down, depressed, or hopeless	0	1	2	3
Trouble falling or staying asleep, or sleeping too much	0	1	2	3
Feeling tired or having little energy	0	1	2	3
Poor appetite or overeating	0	1	2	3
Feeling bad about yourself - or that you are a failure or have let yourself or your family down	0	1	2	3
Trouble concentrating on things, such as reading the newspaper or watching television	0	1	2	3
Moving or speaking so slowly that other people could have noticed? Or the opposite-being so fidgety or restless that you have been moving around a lot more than usual	0	1	2	3
Thoughts that you would be better of dead or of hurting yourself in some way	0	1	2	3

Developer Reference:
Drs. Robert L. Spitzer, Janet B.W. Williams, Kurt Kroenke and colleagues.

Notes

PREGNANCY GUIDE FOR FIRST-TIME DADS

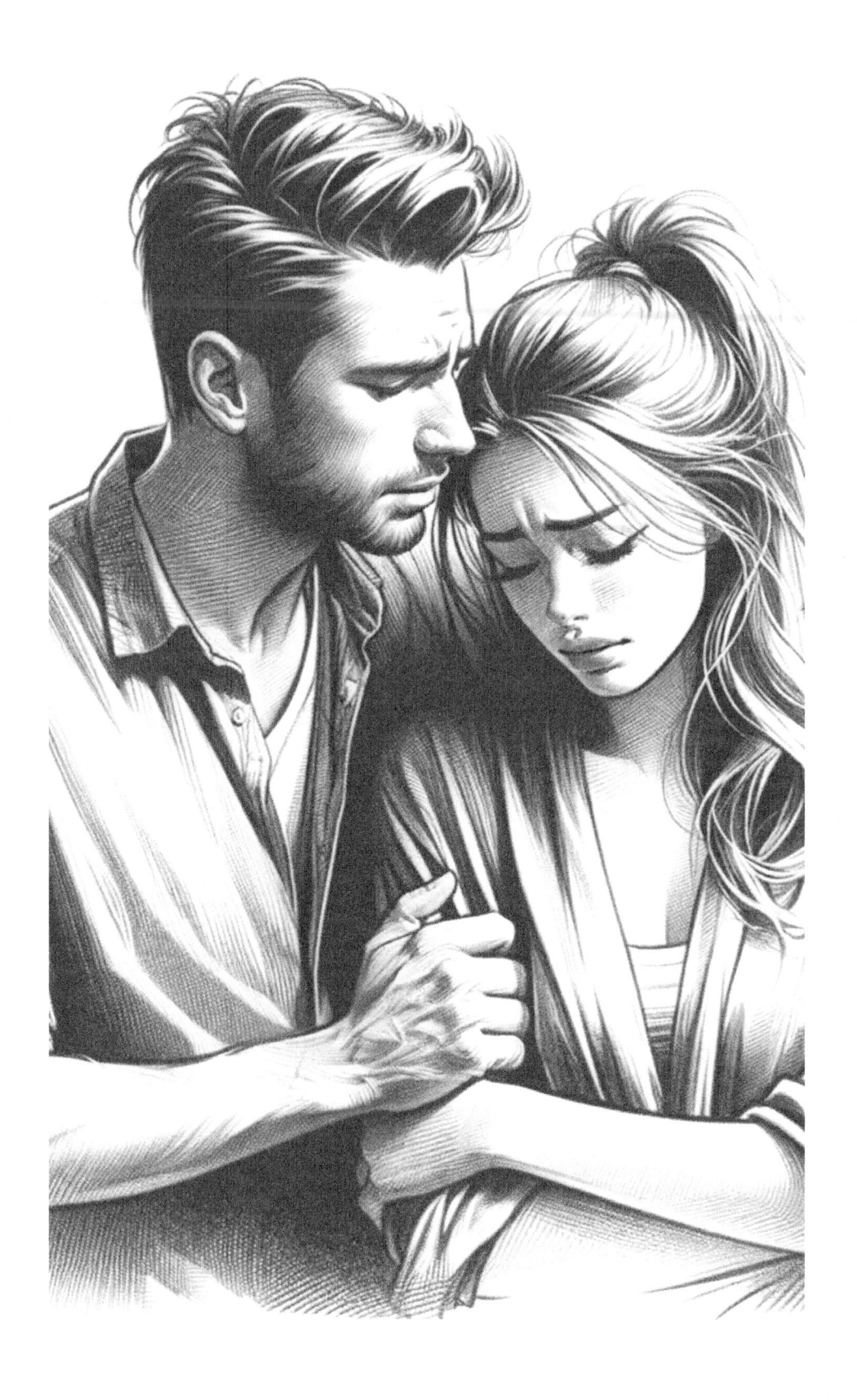

Chapter Eight

Dad by Day, Superhero by Night - Fatherhood in the 21st Century

"The nature of impending fatherhood is that you are doing something that you're unqualified to do, and then you become qualified while doing it."

- John Green

The life of old fathers was quite envy-worthy. According to Anna Machin (2021), an anthropologist studying culture, the duties of old dads were just three things: financial security and providing food; even providing educational support was kind of optional. But, the expectations on today's dads? It's like society wants them to be real-life superheroes, just like the ones we see in movies!

Society is dealing with critical problems right now, and personal experiences and studies point to the role of fathers missing from the public sphere. Young men and women lack male role models: Someone they can respect and want to emulate. And you don't need me to tell you that this has caused severe issues like higher teen pregnancies, divorce rates, substance abuse, and even crimes. The lack of the father's active role reduces children's ability to handle future challenges (Ibrahim et al., 2017).

But wait, there's more... studies upon studies are dropping the bombshell that a father's gestures, actions, word usage, and involvement with children, starting from the early months to the first few years, affect children's intellectual capability, economic achievement, career success, occupational competency, educational expectations, educational attainment, and psychological well-being (Allen & Daly, 2007). Talk about some pressure, right?

That's why the modern role of a father certainly extends beyond just being a breadwinner for the family. Being a dad means being what you wanted in your father. Either your dad was a great role model who taught you how to navigate life, or you wish he were like that. A dad's responsibility remains to be a role model and the anchor children need for guidance. So, let's discuss how to navigate society's and your expectations so you can carve your path as a dad.

MODERN EXPECTATIONS OF THE DAD ROLE

Here's the thing, fellas. In this age of gender equality, we dads are expected to share the responsibility equally with moms when raising our little ones. And hey, if you want to do that, that's a great sentiment! But let's face the facts: Between parental responsibilities, work–family balance, and those hormones, moms still seem to be the MVPs of parenting. Meanwhile, us dads are still trying to figure it all out. But fear not!

Just because we may be less involved doesn't mean we can't rock as role models. Before diving into that though, let's look at the five challenges we fathers face in modern society.

New Fatherhood Identity

Being a dad is like being handed a manual to build our dream spaceship; the problem is that it's written in a language we have never heard of. Besides navigating the unknown, we must deal with the added responsibilities. But hey, at least you are not alone in this adventure!

Drastic Life Changes

Having to do planning in advance before being able to do things you used to do is a significant change for anyone. Society expects us to take all restrictions like that freely with a smile. However, the fact is that there's an adjustment period and feelings of frustration along the way. The adjustment period includes learning how to

- be flexible with your time
- be less spontaneous with plans
- get by with less sleep
- deal with having less time with your partner

The biggest positive is getting your child's love and that you will never run out of funny stories to tell at parties!

But dads need other ways of dealing with their new identity, which society doesn't care much about. So, how can dads deal with this? If you guessed dad communities, you are right on the money!

Chilling With Dad Groups

Meeting with new and older dads is like discovering a secret society, where you realize what's happening to you is not unique. In the dad club, you start to decode the mysteries of fatherhood and settle into what your new identity means. On that note, local dad groups and neighbor families are an excellent way to join this secret society.

Inviting them for a meal at home or outside and then striking up conversations is a good option to introduce yourself. Online communities on social media (e.g., Facebook) are a second option if you can't hit it off with new fathers locally for some reason.

Prioritizing Your Time

Attention, new dads! Just because everyone expects you to be all about the baby and helping mom doesn't mean you must give up everything you love. It's all about setting priorities, my friend.

Sure, you will have less time and might have to let go of a few things. But hey, it's not the end of the world! Take a good look at your schedule and ask yourself, *Do I really need to spend two hours scrolling through social media? Do I need to watch TV every single night? Do I have to hang out with the boys after work every day?* By prioritizing, you will find a way to make things work smoothly and comfortably for your family.

You can be an extra awesome dad when you hold onto some parts of your identity and what matters most to you. Trust me, it will make this whole transition a lot less painful.

Competing Challenges of New Fatherhood

So, as I said, society expects new dads to be pseudo-superheroes. We are expected to earn for the family, maintain a work–life balance, care for the baby, keep the relationship with our spouse strong, and even manage all other relationships. And let's not neglect the ultimate puzzle: figuring out your role as a *dad* during pregnancy and those early months. But hey, don't just wing it and hope for the best!

Relationship Changes

You know how *money matters* can consume your thoughts all day long? Well, baby matters can be just as all-consuming, and it can feel like a tiny dictator has hijacked every chat time. Having a baby in the house means that most, if not all, couple time may suddenly be family time. This also means that you can face a decrease in sexual relations... talk about a tough challenge!

To reclaim some quality time, it's a good idea to revert to the date nights I mentioned before—even if it's just 20 minutes of conversation or a walk outside. Of course, consistency can be a challenge, so get ready for serious logistical planning.

Schedule specific times to discuss babies and other times to put those topics on hold. It's all about finding that delicate balance, one conversation at a time!

Without that balance, when one of you needs to rest for a few days or weeks because of exhaustion, the other can quickly feel like they are doing all the heavy lifting, both literally and figuratively. Without quality time, relationships can resemble a never-ending episode of *Who's on Diaper Duty?* That can lead to extra bickering and relationship deterioration.

Relationships With Friends, Family, and Neighbors

Time becomes a precious commodity, especially in that 1st year. But fear not! Your priority list will be your secret weapon in this.

You can reclaim some of that precious time by requesting your partner to hold down the fort for a bit. Now, it's all about planning and prioritizing like a pro. Remember those epic weekends with friends? Well, now you might have to settle for one day every weekend or maybe even 2 days every fortnight. But hey, it's all worth it!

Also, remember, we have the technology! Embrace the power of video calls to stay connected with those friends you can't visit right now. You can even host gatherings at home while being a dad.

And if you need a breather, don't hesitate to call in reinforcements. Ask a relative or a friend to hold down the fort while you sneak away for a little hangout time. And when it comes to family, get creative! Take the baby on a ride to visit close relatives or invite them to take care of the baby.

Believe me, if you are determined to make those relationships work, you will find a way to make it happen.

Bonding With Baby

Ever heard of skin-to-skin contact? It's like a secret handshake with babies. While moms have had a head start with that direct connection through pregnancy and breastfeeding, we dads can still build those strong bonds.

Sure, we might not get as much time off work, but who needs sleep anyway, right? (pun intended). Considering our late start, let's ignore society's unrealistic expectations and give ourselves some extra time. Maybe it will take a few months or even a year, but we will get there and create a deep bond with our little one!

Negative Feelings and Fears

Being a dad is a role that's so vague that even the most experienced dads can feel lost about how to manage their time. And I can't forget the lack of reliable sources for dad's knowledge. How are dads supposed to know how to help their partner or soothe their baby when most information is as clear as mud?

The uncertainty of how to stay involved naturally creates worries and anxiety. Dads start questioning themselves and doubting their abilities. These doubts then make dads unable to perform at their best, creating a never-ending cycle of negative feelings.

But, dear dads! Embrace the chaos, learn as you go, and remember that a little humor goes a long way.

My first trip with a baby was a comedy of errors. I had packed everything I could possibly think of, but in my haste, I overlooked one crucial detail: diapers. You know where this is going, don't you? There I was, in the middle of a crowded mall, with my son having an explosive diaper situation, and me without a single diaper in sight. Let's just say I've never hustled to a store faster in my life. That day, I not only embraced my role as a modern dad, but I also became a diaper bag aficionado.

Parenting Anxiety

To combat the lack of knowledge, we need to gather knowledge! Simple, right? Now, while there may be fewer resources for dads, it's not like there are none.

Dads need at least a rough game plan of how they plan to proceed and basic knowledge of things for that. For example, babies start

- crawling within 6 to 10 months.
- uttering some words around the year mark.
- requiring potty training at the 2-year mark.
- drawing shapes around the 2-year mark.

And so on. It's essential to inform ourselves about parenting milestones related to baby development. Think of it as our superpower! Knowing the monthly milestones and what we can do to achieve them can help us understand what to expect and what we can do to support our partner and baby.

However, nothing will ever fully prepare you for the challenges that being a dad throws at you. But just like how knowing the exam process beforehand can help you be more flexible with your time management and prioritization in stressful moments, knowing milestones and planning around them will help you be flexible as a dad.

Managing the Emotional Fuel Tank

It's not all smooth sailing sometimes. Unexpected things pop up from time to time, and you may find yourself needing to adjust your life faster than a diaper change. Now, I know time management can be a real challenge. Between changing diapers, feeding, and trying to catch some shut-eye, it's easy to feel you don't have enough time. Sometimes, that can end up with you feeling like you have never seen personal, family, and relationship time before.

This may create frustration, which can lead to interesting coping mechanisms like smoking, alcohol, working long hours, listening to music, and other activities. But fear not, I have got some tips to help you navigate this without resorting to becoming an alcoholic, a workaholic, or a one-man band!

Coping With Stress

First things first, don't be too hard on yourself. Mistakes happen, and that's okay!

Society might have some crazy expectations, but remember, you are human too. So, put down that pack of cigarettes, step away from the bottle, and explore healthier alternatives.

One of the best ways to find relief is by keeping your friends and spouse close. Don't be afraid to ask for help from your close social network; they are there for a reason! And when things get overwhelming, it's time to call in the reinforcements. Yes, I am talking about those creatures called babysitters. They can give you some much-needed time to recharge and reset.

But here's the real secret: It's not just about external solutions. It's about challenging those pesky thoughts in your mind. You know, the ones that say you are making too many mistakes or that you are never doing enough. Trust me, those thoughts are as helpful as a soggy diaper.

So, take a deep breath, remind yourself you are doing your best, and let go of those unrealistic expectations.

Taking care of your mind is taking care of yourself. Time management also plays a big role in that. Set realistic expectations, prioritize what's important, and don't forget to give yourself a pat on the back now and then.

But, my friend, if you find yourself stuck in a never-ending loop of frustration and things aren't improving for weeks, don't hesitate to reach out to therapists—they are like the superheroes of the mind. They can help you get unstuck and back on track.

Lack of Support

Let's take a moment to appreciate the plight of new dads. They are expected to do a million things, but where's the support? It's like they are searching for a mythical creature called Dad Support that no one seems to have seen!

Even doctors seem to be in on the conspiracy. They put all the focus on mom, leaving poor dads on the sidelines. It's like they're saying, "Hey, Dad, figure it out on your own!" And how can we forget about the workplace? Trying to get some time off can feel like climbing Mount Everest!

But here's the kicker: When dads stay silent, everyone assumes we have everything under control. Just like with superheroes! Now, we don't want pity, but a little support and guidance wouldn't hurt, right? So, let's solve this dilemma together!

Loneliness and Isolation

Transitioning into parenthood can leave dads feeling like they are on a different planet from their friends, partners, and even themselves, and there's no means of communication. But don't panic! The key to surviving this adventure is embracing change and adapting like a chameleon.

Pro Tip:

Don't be afraid to ask for help. I know, I know, it goes against our *I can handle anything* instincts, but sometimes we need backup. Reach out to your relatives or friends and let them lend a hand. Trust me, they won't be able to read your mind (unless they have superpowers we don't know about), so it's up to us to speak up and ask for that much-needed assistance.

And hey, don't forget about your fellow new dads! They are like your partners in crime, except the crime is changing diapers, and the getaway car is a stroller. They are going through the same ups and downs and sleepless nights, so connect with them, share your hilarious poop explosion stories, and lean on each other for emotional support. Remind yourself that you are not alone in this.

Sure, it can feel a bit lonely at times, but thinking that no one is there to help is like trying to build a sandcastle in the middle of the desert. It's just not gonna work. So, let's make the effort to break down those walls and let others in. Trust me, it will make a big difference.

REDEFINING FATHERHOOD: CREATING YOUR NARRATIVE

Now, let's break down the fatherhood narrative. It's as simple as sticking to a healthy diet and hitting the gym to get fit. Simple, but it takes some discipline. And guess what? You can start being a role model from the moment your baby is just weeks old. It's never too early to start!

So, here's your game plan for creating your path ahead. Pay attention, new dads, because these four things are your secret weapons to fatherhood success!

Treating Your Partner and Relationships With Respect

Being a dad can feel like directing a silent-comedy drama for your kids. They may not always understand what you say, but they definitely observe what you do.

Ensure you are not dealing with people angrily or making fun of them behind their backs in front of kids. Kids are like little detectives. They see and absorb everything, especially how you treat their mom. That's why keeping the household free from constant fighting and bickering is essential, as it takes a toll on their mental health.

Now, I'm not saying you can't disagree with that quirky relative or have a little spat with your spouse now and then—that's just part of life. But what you can't do is let your kids be aware of all the drama, even if it's happening.

Remember, you are the director of the family comedy show, so let's keep it light, funny, and drama-free!

Getting to Know Your Kids

From the moment they are in the womb until they hit their teenage years, you need to spend time getting to know your kids. Learn about the new things they have learned, new hobbies, new moves, what they like, what they are afraid of, how they deal with their emotions, and so on.

When they are a little older, navigating the path of fatherhood involves creating a safe space for your kids to open up to you, which is only possible when you make them feel that you won't overreact. Trust me, once, there was this fantastic dad who was pretty calm most of the time, but one day, he lost it when his little daughter mentioned a boy's name with a smile!

Turns out, it was just a harmless joke, and the girl never even brought up the boy again! So, yes, sometimes we dads can't help but overreact, but hey, that's where the mom swoops in to save the day!

Letting Your Kids Know You

Children are little detectives, always curious about the world around them. So, why not use their curiosity to your advantage and become the ultimate dad hero in their eyes? Share your stories with them (even when they are a few weeks old), and watch as you become their inspiration and guide for life.

These stories will help their development in the starting weeks and months. And when they are a little older, stories will be carried with them throughout their lives, shaping their decisions and filling them with wonder. Not only does this create a deeper bond with your baby, but it will also help you connect with them emotionally.

You can tap into the baby's curiosity in so many fun ways! Take them to a soccer game or a museum, or embark on a short family picnic adventure with mom. The possibilities are many!

Knowing the Science Behind Things

I say that because without proper knowledge that we can put our two cents on, most dads stay in a reactionary state regarding parenting. New dads whose dads were strict may end up spoiling their kids, and new dads whose dads ended up making them spoiled may end up enforcing excess discipline.

Learning about the development milestones is a great way to know what to do. But hey, here's what the bigger picture is like.

Think of yourself as a nurse, except you are a nurse with a sense of humor. Treat those little ones like mini ICU patients until they are about 7 years old. Show them kindness, and they will learn kindness. Just be careful not to turn them into game, snack, or show addicts. You only have until they are around 12 to maintain some control, so buckle up! After that, you will ride shotgun in their life, hoping you taught them well enough.

I know of a dad who built 11 branches of his business, but he realized he messed up when he saw his daughter bringing back boys who only cared about complimenting her to get what they wanted. Poor guy just broke down crying. That's why spending time with kids, aka managing work–life balance, is a must, and we will dive into that in the next chapter.

Notes

PREGNANCY GUIDE FOR FIRST-TIME DADS

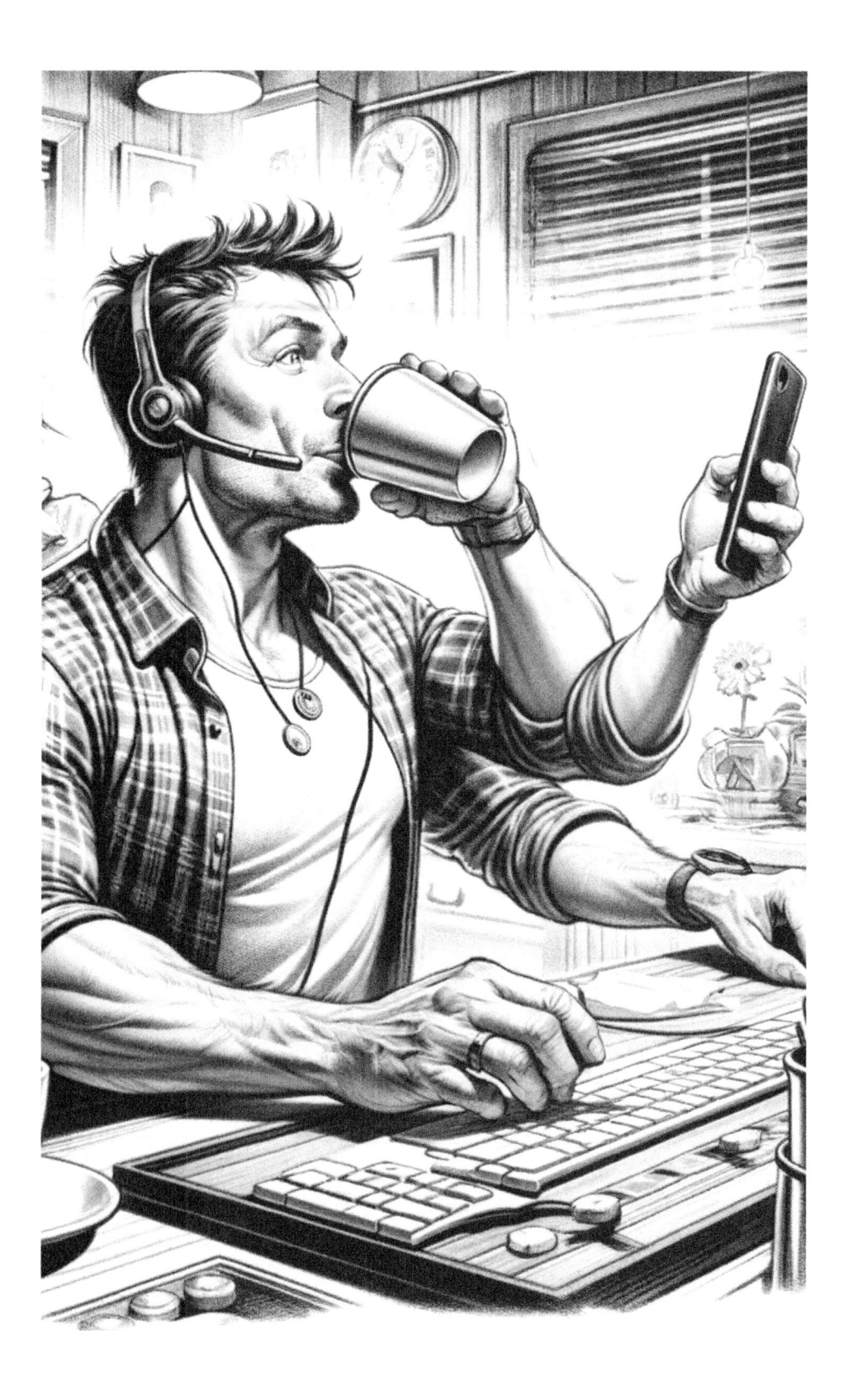

Chapter Nine

Coffee, Conference Calls, and Cuddles - The Modern Dad's Trifecta

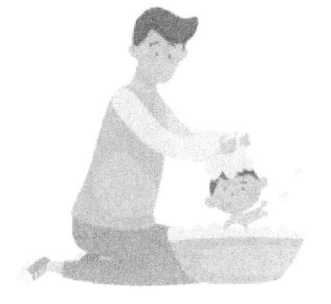

> "You can't truly be considered successful in your business life if your home life is in shambles."
> - Zig Ziglar

When you think about balance, what pops into your mind? Well, some things that come to mind may include the metaphorical balance between good and evil, the right mix for the perfect dish, and the balance of justice where we give equal attention to both sides!

But, my fellow new dads, here's the deal: Work–life balance is not some epic battle where you win by defeating a supervillain once or a courtroom drama where you always have to be perfectly fair. No, no, no!

Work–life balance is more like an ongoing puzzle you constantly try to solve. There will be moments when you are swamped with extra work at the office, home, or both, all while running on less sleep than you would like. But fear not! With a little planning, a couple of cups of coffee (or two), and a focus on the little things, you will navigate this balancing act like a pro.

WHY WORK-LIFE BALANCE IS A DIFFERENT KIND OF BALANCING

I once found myself in an important Zoom meeting with a pacifier in my mouth and a baby in my arms, trying to 'shush' him while discussing quarterly projections. Apparently, pacifiers don't mute dads on Zoom calls, who knew?

You see, we don't get to choose when urgent work situations pop up, demanding all-nighters. And we don't get to decide when Mom suddenly needs you at home or the baby has a doctor's appointment. It's like life has a secret agenda to keep us on our toes.

Following a strict routine of separating work time and home time can feel like trying to catch a greased pig!

Now, you have a leg up on the balance game if you are a freelancer. You can twist and turn your 24/7 schedule like a yoga master. Meanwhile, business owners and 9-to-5ers can find it a bit trickier to find that sweet spot. But don't fret yet, my fellas, because I have some gloves to help you wrangle that elusive greased pig!

Opposing Needs

Because of gender equality, we want to be high achievers in both our careers and homes. We dream of climbing the corporate ladder while building a solid bond with our little ones. It's like wanting to be Elon Musk at work and Mr. Mom at home.

But here's the catch—there's only so much time and energy in a day. You can't magically create 28 hours, no matter how much you wish. However, there is some good news for you, my friend.

While you can't add more hours to the day, you can undoubtedly increase your productivity during those precious hours.

Sure, sometimes you may not have more than an hour or two a day to spend with your family, but you can make those hours count! You can do that by focusing on quality over quantity. Your loved ones will appreciate your undivided attention, even if you occasionally need to work long hours or a crazy week.

Trying to force a schedule that gives you 4 hours of family time while constantly glancing at your device, checking emails, or making work calls is a recipe for disaster.

Trust me, your family won't be thrilled with that approach. So, embrace the limited time you have and make it count!

Difficulty in Maintaining Quality Time

Did you know that current dads are spending about three times more time with their kids? (Livingston & Parker, 2019). But here's the scary part: Are we really spending quality time like the old dads?

I mean, let's be honest: We are all guilty of using our phones, especially social media, even when we are *spending time together.* We could be sitting on the couch, watching a movie, or having a meal together, but our eyes constantly shift to our screens. Can we really call that *quality time?*

And let's keep in mind how social media messes with our perception of time. We might think we are spending a couple of hours with our partner, but in reality, it's more like 20 or 30 minutes. Each notification or interaction with mobile distracts and diverts the focus for some time (Stothart et al., 2015). Not to mention, we can end up back on the phone before our minds can refocus on our family.

If you know someone who has tried a mobile detox, ask them how time seems to slow down for them. Even 30 minutes can feel like an eternity when you are not constantly reaching for your phone.

Having a mobile device at our fingertips all the time takes away from those precious moments of slowness that we crave. So, when you are with your family, resist the urge to use your phone. Whether eating, cooking, watching a movie, chatting, or playing with your partner, let's make a pact to put away emails, work-related phone calls, and social media.

It might seem challenging, but we can make it happen with some prioritization!

INTEGRATING WORK AND LIFE

Integrating work with life deals with five things:

1. Being realistic about expectations
2. Doing a resource analysis and performing prioritization
3. Making goals based on priorities
4. Using longer time slots and conveying boundaries
5. Focusing on the little things

Being Realistic About Work–Life Balance

They say that knowing there's a problem is the first step to creating a solution. As a new dad, it's in our best interest to admit that your life is now different and *needs some changes*. Forget about the mindset of a corporate warrior who works overtime and climbs the corporate ladder at rocket speed.

You are a man with a new set of emotions and changed priorities.

Your ambitious to-do list may now include a 30-minute nap instead of an extra 30-minute cold email outreach. Instead of giving 200% like you used to, save some of that energy for your family. You only have so much time and energy.

This is another reason why being part of communities with fellow new dads navigating this journey is essential. They can help set realistic expectations and remind you that you are not alone in going through changes. It's comforting to validate your experiences and know you are not going off track. This can work wonders in making you feel more in control.

So, acknowledge your new situation and feelings, and watch yourself and your confidence grow!

Thinking Holistically

A realistic work–life balance is not just a never-ending cycle of work, family, work, family! You have needs beyond that: emotional, spiritual, physical, and intellectual needs. Taking care of all of them is key for any long-term strategy.

Let me tell you a story about a woman working 10 hours daily and commuting 2 hours a day. She felt like she couldn't make her relationships work. But then she read a book on work–life balance and decided to change. Can you guess what she did?

She started going to the gym for 1 to 2 hours daily! Lady, that's not how things are done! Don't get me wrong, taking care of health is excellent, but this was just a bit extreme, don't you think?

You see, some things have higher priority than others. Physical health is good, but meaningful relationships are a must to have a healthy emotional state. If the lady just spent 15 minutes on stretching exercises and the rest of the 1–2 hours connecting with people, she would be in a way wholesome position! Let's look at work-life balance holistically and consider six factors:

- **Work:** This includes all things work-related.

- **Social:** This involves family, parents, relatives, friends, neighbors, and colleagues.

- **Personal Development:** Taking care of your physical health and developing new skills.

- **Relaxation:** Making time for activities that help you unwind, like some good old dad time.

- **Spiritual:** This includes religious prayers or meditation, something you find inner peace with.

- **Sleep:** Not forgetting the importance of a good night's sleep and some afternoon naps.

And just like the example of the lady taught us, we need to first learn about our *priorities* and then create new habits based on them.

Juggling With Prioritization

As a dad, you will need to make a ton of trade-offs along the dad journey, just like in the corporate world. For that, let's first start with a resource analysis, dad-style. How much time and energy do you have each day? Once you have got that cleared up, rank your repeating tasks by their importance. You can use a super simple rating scale (like your gut feeling) or a complicated one (like decision matrices) to rank your priorities in the six categories above.

But watch out for those sneaky fake priorities! They are worse than an underhanded employee trying to steal office supplies!

Fake vs. Real Priorities

Work can sometimes be rightfully urgent. But let's face it, most of the time, it's more like a slow crawl than a sprint. So, when you rush to your family, only to eat dinner alone and drown in a sea of emails, you should better realize that you are falling victim to the *artificial urgency* syndrome.

I mean, what's the worst that could happen if you checked them tomorrow? When prioritizing, it's good to ask yourself critical questions, like, *Would the world end if I left those emails for another day?*

Trust me, new dads, avoiding artificial urgency is the key to maintaining your sanity and being present for the ones who matter most.

Pro Tip:

Try a digital detox for 12 to 48 hours on a weekend. You can start with 12 hours and increase it now and then. It's a proven way to get past the *artificial urgency* syndrome related to technology.

Squeezing More Time by Optimizing Your Routine

It's crucial to optimize your day by staying healthy and getting up early—earlier than your partner and the rest of the world. Why? Well, it's like you are a secret agent, but you are saving your sanity instead of the world!

In the morning, you can use your focused energy on work or family matters and plan your day without distractions. It's like having your superhero mode activated! Optimizing your day will increase your overall time and energy, and you can avoid having to cross out those extra one or two things you actually like from your to-do list.

Trust me, your body and mind work better on this schedule. It's like all those famous quotes about mornings were written just for you!

Now, if you don't already have this schedule, make it another one of your goals. Think of it as a boot camp to prep for those sleepless nights ahead. It's a time that forces you to be comfortable being uncomfortable. So, new dads, get ready to optimize your day, embrace the early mornings, and conquer the world (or at least your to-do list).

Setting Goals

Knowing what you can do puts you in a better position to make your action plan. Let's break it down into six categories and set some goals, shall we?

- **Work goals:** Crush those key performance indicators for the next 3 months!

- **Social goals:** Prepare morning meals for myself and my spouse, help with the house chores for 1 hour in the evening, do an activity with my partner for 1 hour after the evenings, and go outside on weekends.

- **Personal development goals:** Get my blood pumping with a morning gym routine, fuel my body with healthy meals at regular times, read or listen to my pregnancy book for 15 minutes daily, and dive into that artificial intelligence course for 30 minutes on weekend afternoons.

- **Relaxation:** Unwind in the evening with a 30-minute breathing exercise, de-stress with 2 hours of TV time on weekends, and an extra 10-minute shower every other day.

- **Spiritual:** Calm my inner self by performing religious prayers at their designated times, doing introspection (analyzing my thoughts) or retrospection (analyzing my routine) for 30 minutes in the evening.

- **Sleep:** A solid 8-hour snooze from 10 p.m. to wake up early at 6 a.m., and a 30-minute afternoon nap.

Why Is That Important?

Now, I know it might seem like a lot of paperwork to do all at once, but don't worry! Take it one step at a time, spread it out over a few weeks, and dedicate just a few tens of minutes each day.

Remember, if you don't plan your life, someone else will plan it for you—that someone can be your employer or somebody else.

Here's the fun part: You won't always meet every goal, and that's okay! Life happens, and goals are meant to be flexible. The important thing is that you are giving yourself direction and clarity by setting goals.

You will also become more mindful (selective) of how you spend your time. So, next time you come across something tempting like a captivating news story, an intriguing Medium question, or a flashy advertisement, ask yourself if it truly matters to you and if you need to check it. This little reality check will often help you stay on track.

Trust me, the method of setting goals has been tried and tested by many people. So, embrace the power of goal-setting, and let's make your dad life even more awesome!

Dividing Your Time

If the world were ideal, then a perfect routine like 9 a.m.–5 p.m., work; 5 p.m.–7 p.m., me time; and 7 p.m.–10 p.m., family time, would definitely work! But we new dads don't live in an ideal world. Sometimes, we are needed at work, and sometimes, we are required at home.

So, if we try to make schedules the normal way, we can end up adjusting them a million times! And trust me, that can make anyone exhausted and disoriented.

However, here's a little secret that has worked for many: setting boundaries. Now, I know it can be challenging, especially when juggling a job or business and family life. But don't worry. No matter your work situation, it's not a hopeless cause. You can still set some broad boundaries, which will make a big difference.

Setting Boundaries

Time slots are like the superhero capes of productivity! Picture this: You work a 6-hour slot, then take a well-deserved 90-minute break slot. No work-related stuff is allowed during that break! Just like that, setting boundaries in the workplace to maintain your planned slots is the secret trick.

If you have colleagues who constantly bug you after work, let them know you are off the grid for emails during nonworking hours.

You can even request your boss to give you that flexibility. And if they don't give you the green light, it might be time to find a ship that sails in your favor. Trust me, there are plenty out there!

Now, you can be the boundary-setting champion if you are a high-level executive! Lead by example and create a culture where people can focus on their family in family time without interruptions. That also means resisting the urge to send or respond to emails after your designated time.

But wait, there's more to this! Family time can also have its time slots.

How about a 1-hour slot where you tackle household chores and errands together? It's like a chore-busting hour! And then, reserve a glorious 2-hour slot where you stash your phone out of sight and fully engage with your partner and baby. It's like a digital detox for quality family time.

Divide and conquer, my friend! By organizing your time into slots, you can tackle multiple tasks in one go and save yourself from the headache of overthinking every little thing. Time slots are like magic. Even if you take a quick 10-minute restroom break or chat with a colleague for 5 minutes, commit to finishing that 6-hour work slot without going overboard or falling short, and you may be amazed at how much you can accomplish!

What About the Days With Extra Work

As a dad, there will be days when work demands more of your attention. But hey, here's a tip: Try fitting work time around family time, not the other way around. If you find yourself at home with a work to-do list, you can do these things:

- Make the most of those precious afternoon naps when the mom (or baby) catches some z's.

- Hit the bed early and tackle the extra work in the morning.

- If the newborn hits the snooze button early, seize that golden opportunity to leap into some extra tasks.

And on those super busy days during and after pregnancy, consider sending Mom and Baby on a well-deserved evening out or to visit the grandparents and relatives.

Here's the best part: Even if things don't go according to plan sometimes, trust me, your family won't mind the occasional long days.

Become More Creative With Time

Want to reclaim some precious time as a new dad? Embrace your inner laziness and automate things! Say goodbye to bill-payment hassles by setting up automatic payments, and let Amazon do the shipping for you instead of you sightseeing the stores.

Embrace your inner time-saving miser and use that extra time to focus on the little everyday things that matter most!

Become Part of the 5 a.m. Club

Sleeping early and waking up early is the cheat code of productivity. It's like getting more hours in your day. When you have made 6 a.m. your habit, and it's easy to commit, you should start waking up a bit earlier and move yourself to the 5 a.m. club. Don't forget to start over and sharpen your schedule after that.

Now, there's an ambitious goal that only a select few of the first-time Jedi dads can achieve—being a part of the 4 a.m. club. Now those are goals! Getting up earlier is the only actual way to gain more time in life. The early bird truly gets the worm.

Tip 1:

Try this schedule together with an afternoon nap of 30 minutes. The body tends to get tired about 8 hours after waking up, and a short nap can give the much-needed rest.

Tip 2:

Try the 5 a.m. routine in weeks of less work. The body can take a few days to adjust to a new sleep routine. Also, don't force the 4 a.m. waking up routine if your schedule doesn't allow it—like if you frequently sleep late (after 9 p.m. or 10 p.m.) or can't take afternoon naps.

Keep That Coffee Mug Close

We must master the art of going by on less sleep in our daily lives. Coffee mugs are your best friends to do that. Coffee in the morning and afternoon can give you the energy to brave the day. Just don't drink coffee at night, except if you want to go without sleep.

Use the Little Things

Alright, new dads. You have big dreams of taking your little one and partner to amusement parks every month or even going all out and hitting another city for their birthday. Not wrong goals, but let's aim higher, shall we? Your kids and partner need more than special occasions and vacations to feel love.

Spending Quality Time With Your Family

Quality time with your newborn kid is when you stumble out of bed in the morning and take a refreshing walk around the neighborhood, taking the baby in the stroller. Quality time is when you brave the chaotic nature of baby potty and vomit, and burp them while carrying them. Quality time is when you become the master storyteller and keep telling them stories, even though they can only respond with staring and the occasional smile.

In the same way, quality time with your partner is when you take her to a park in the evening, even if it's just to watch the ducks waddle around. Quality time is when you show care by cooking a special homemade meal together on a random day (or on weekends). And don't forget those late-night chats before sleep, where you discuss everything from the meaning of life to the latest Netflix binge.

Fellas, remember, quality time is a lot about those little moments—because they create a significant impact. So, embrace the day-to-day interactions and give importance to the minor details. And trust me, paying attention to the details can be pretty darn satisfying when it's your little one or partner.

FINAL TIPS

I have seen all kinds of dads in different situations. Some were jet-setting (traveling a lot) for work, while others worked from their couches. A job requiring occasional week (or month) long travel or extra hours can still work. After all, even superheroes have to go on missions! But if you have the choice between two similar jobs, it's best to pick one that keeps you close to your family and gives you flexibility with your time.

The overriding theme in all situations is that dads must be intentional parents, prioritizing their family and other commitments. They need to plan and make deliberate decisions all the time, actively. The result? A fulfilling life as both a parent and a professional in their field.

With that finished, we are ready to move on to welcoming that baby into the world! Let's explore that together in the following two chapters!

Notes

TAYLOR ANTHONY

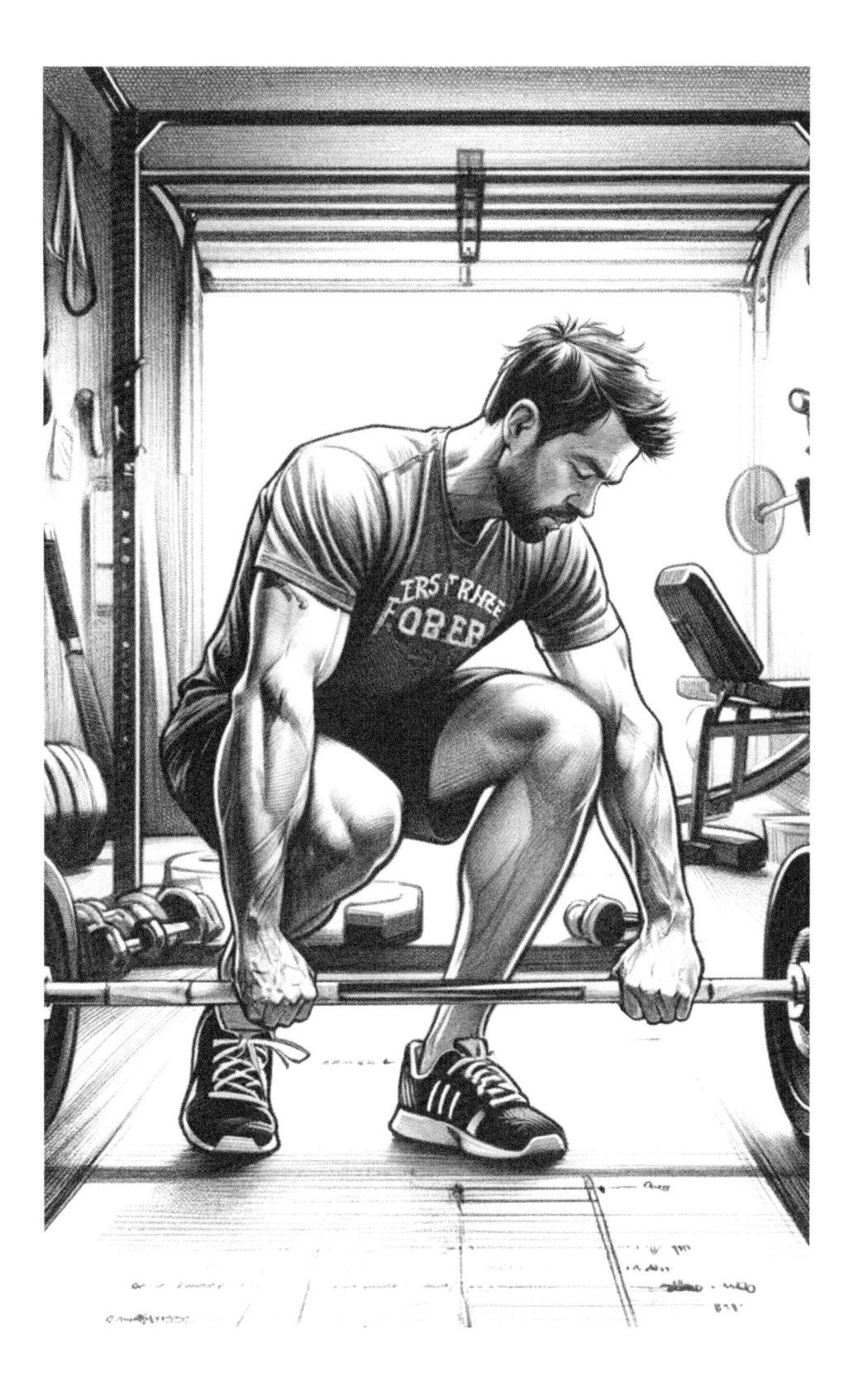

Chapter Ten

Womb Whisperer - My Journey to Becoming Baby's First Friend

"The most important thing in the world is family and love."

- John Wooden

It's time to address a burning question: Is it worth connecting with your unborn star as a new dad?

I mean, we are already dealing with mama changes, personal commitments, and workplace adjustments, so why bother when they can't even respond, right? Well, not really.

You may have noticed with your friends or relatives that babies are usually more attached to mothers than fathers.

Remember when we talked about the baby's ear developing in the second trimester? That means, while mom is chatting with her friends or complaining about that back pain to grandma, the baby is listening and getting familiar with her voice!

Adding to that, a fetus can sense the emotional state of their mother, and their growth is affected by the emotional changes: fetal activity, heartbeats, sleep patterns, and movement are all affected by emotional changes in mom like long-term stress and anxiety (Kinsella & Monk, 2009). This means the baby is getting familiar with the mom's body throughout pregnancy.

This also means the baby is starting from a clean slate only when it comes to dad! But don't worry, I have got tips to help you navigate that hurdle. Sure, the baby may start with kicks and posture changes, but they will definitely respond to you!

BUDDING THE BOND

Since you are eager to become the baby's BFF (best father forever), there are plenty of ways to make that happen. But before we dive into activities like baby talk and gentle pats, we need to free up some resources, don't you think?

Focus on Your Mental Health

Now, here's a little roadblock that can get in the way of you and your unborn baby becoming best buds: Dealing with stress and work-life balance issues. Don't worry; we have tackled those things! In Chapter 9, we covered a bunch of ways to help you juggle your work and family time like a pro. And hey, we even dived into how to handle those mental roller-coasters of pregnancy throughout this book. So, make sure to put those tips into action and free up some precious time and energy for your baby.

Particularly, don't forget to plan your finances with a budget and have a good old chat with your spouse when needed. Trust me, you don't want to be stuck worrying about money all the time. Remember, you may feel like you are not quite up to building this bond without time and energy.

Work Together With Your Spouse

When the mom gets hit with the nesting urge, you may not even realize it until most of the baby preparations are over! Don't let mom tackle all the preparations alone.

Let her know you are ready to be her partner in parenthood. This includes shopping for baby items, decorating and painting the baby's room, setting up the crib, deciding baby names, installing the baby car seat, cleaning the baby's room, and everything else under the roof. Spending time like this builds excitement for the new baby and creates precious moments with the mom, starting from the first trimester.

Remember, building a solid bond with your baby involves teamwork. So, my friend, roll up those sleeves and put that baby crib where it belongs!

Going Together With Her on Appointments

Trying to picture your baby's looks can be like solving a mystery. But joining your partner on ultrasound days is like getting a secret clue through an insider source.

Suddenly, that little imaginary bean becomes a real life in your mind! And hey, if you want to keep the ultrasound picture (also called a sonogram) on your phone or desk, you can go for it.

Aside from the ultrasounds, attending other appointments and asking questions is like being a detective on a mission. You are not just building anticipation in yourself for your child. You are also giving your partner some superb backup.

So, grab your magnifying glass and go with her on appointments.

Options in Your Tool Set

The secret recipe to bond with your unborn one is: Talking to them, buying some stuff, and giving gentle tummy pats. It's like a magical spell that will make your heart melt.

Talking to Them

In case you were wondering, babies don't know what we are blabbering about. But hey, that doesn't mean there can't be some benefits, right?

The key here is to familiarize them with our voice, just like the momma. You can start with some daily rituals, like *hello* in the morning, *goodbye* when you head off to work, *I am back* when you return home, or simply sharing the thrilling details of your day. This little trick will pay off when you need to comfort them during those (inevitable) crying sessions.

That's because your voice will give them a sense of familiarity and safety, second only to the mom! So, it's like saving yourself a ton of trouble without even realizing it!

Reading to Them

Alright, chatting away with a tiny human who doesn't respond the way we want can be a bit exhausting. But fear not! There's a clever workaround: reading to your little one.

Yup, you heard me right!

You can grab a storybook, your all-time favorite novel, an interesting article, or anything else that tickles your fancy. Hey, you can even read out hilarious memes and add your witty comments. The important thing is that your baby gets to hear your fantastic voice!

Singing to Them

Sing to your baby all you want, even if your spouse raises some eyebrows at your voice! The good news is that your little one won't mind at all! Lullabies like "Twinkle Twinkle, Little Star" are a fantastic option because they have a soothing effect on unborn babies, and you can usually feel that by patting the tummy.

There's a bonus: Your baby will likely recognize the lullaby even after birth, which will help them feel safe and peaceful when they listen to it in the future. So, go ahead and sing away—it may be an excellent way to capture their attention after pregnancy.

Tip:

A good way to keep the routine is to talk or sing to them at bedtime.

Note:

Heavy or loud music, like rock music, can be stressful for the baby's sensitive ears, so steer away from stuff like that.

Introducing Baby to Relatives

On the phone with relatives? Get the baby on call, too. It's like a conference call to introduce the baby to Grandpa and Grandma and other relatives. It is a great way to connect with family and familiarize the baby with their voices.

Patting the Tummy

Patting the tummy can be a satisfying experience throughout the pregnancy, but it becomes much more interesting in the last few months. Your little one will sometimes surprise you by responding to your tummy pats with kicks, punches, or posture changes. It then becomes like a mysterious game of "Guess the Body Part," is it a hand, a knee, or a foot?

And here's a mind-blowing fact: While babies may not understand our words and actions just yet, it seems they have a sixth sense for detecting emotions. Research shows that babies born with gentle tummy pats have almost twice as much chance of having a calm and easygoing temper, and lower negative moods (Wang et al., 2015). So, new dads, shower them with love and create a sense of trust and safety with gentle baby pats, soft lullabies, and warm words.

Tip:

You can hang out with your partner every evening to participate in this sport.

Taking Memorable Notes and Splurging a Little

Buying or setting up small things like pampers, cribs, baby car seats, baby feeders, and other items is an excellent way to start the bond with the baby. But why stop there?

We dads love to imagine all the fun activities we will do when they are a little older, so you should take it to the next level if your budget allows. Go ahead and splurge a little on that small fishing pole, the hand-sized football, or anything else that pops into your mind. It's like cementing those future adventures in our minds and making them more tangible to us—remember not to go overboard!

And here's another thing: Why not write down these thoughts and feelings you are having in notes? It's a great way to calm down and root out negative thoughts. You can even imagine sharing them with the baby in the near future.

Imagine their reaction when they read about all the fantastic plans you had for them even before they were born!

One tip to remember when bonding with the baby through your voice, tummy pats, and other interactions is to try a routine. Building a routine will help you stay consistent and can help the baby adapt to you and your partner's lifestyle. For example, let's say your partner takes a bath before bedtime. You can make it a habit to talk to the baby after that shower. Who knows, it may help the baby understand it's time to wind down and reduce the chances of the baby throwing a dance party in the middle of the night!

With that finished, the next chapter contains a crash course to help you navigate the months right after the baby's birth. Let's move!

Notes

PREGNANCY GUIDE FOR FIRST-TIME DADS

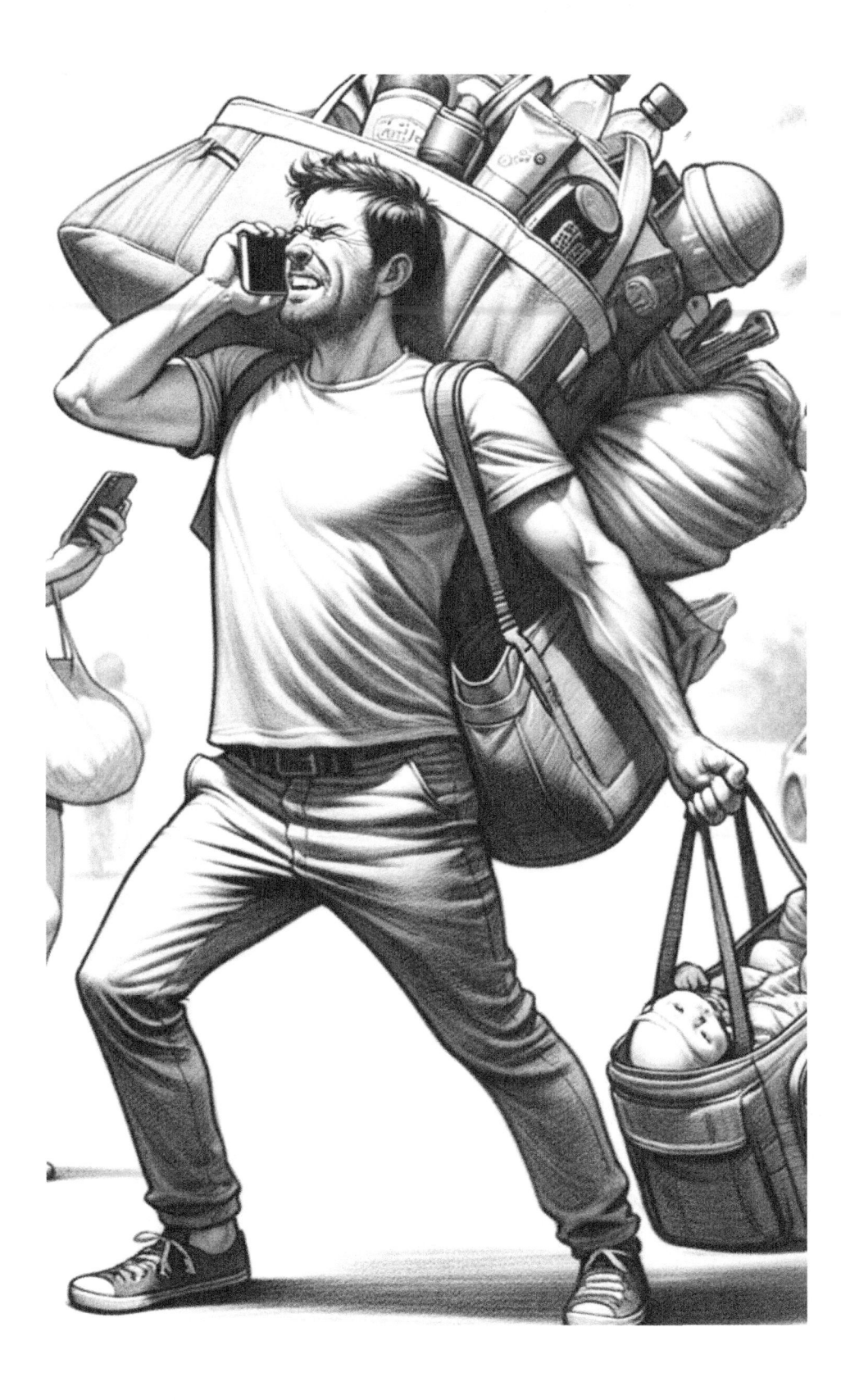

Chapter Eleven

Surviving Baby Boot Camp - Becoming a Pro Dad

"Every father should remember one day his son will follow his example, not his advice."

— Charles Kettering

You should hopefully have a little extra time and energy on your hands if you followed most of the tips I mentioned consistently.

Now, the question is what to do with that newfound vigor. Well, you can do many things, except participating in breastfeeding, save that for your little one.

Firstly, you will be able to learn much about your little bundle of joy. From washing them, changing diapers, putting them to sleep, and even mastering the art of burping, you will climb the ladder to become a pro in no time.

And let's not forget about the precious resource of sleep! You can create a rough schedule to maximize those elusive z's. Just remember, as a new dad, you must become a walking, talking, chore-handling machine yourself. If you weren't much of a household chores expert before, don't worry! Feel free to ask for assistance in learning them from relatives and your partner as soon as possible.

Alternatively, if you and your partner are working outside and planning for a nanny, you can hire one who will also help with some household chores. But even if you hire a nanny, dedicate time for childcare in some way to build a bond with the baby.

Now, here's the deal: Even though you don't have this issue, some dads can feel a bit hesitant about bonding and getting involved in childcare. Society has a funny way of ingraining the idea that only moms can be the *actual caregivers*. This happens because of reasons like people showing this attitude unconsciously, the workplace giving less off-time to fathers, and people only telling mothers *what to do.* It's like they think dads are just there for comic relief!

But fear not, my friend, because you have plenty of ways to be involved and develop that special bond with your little one. In fact, it's highly recommended for many reasons that we will explore soon. So, let's dive in and discover the joys of being a hands-on dad!

IMPORTANCE OF DEVELOPING A BOND WITH THE BABY

Babies are incredibly dependent on parents, and their brains go through a lot of development and neuron pruning during this time. Just think about it: They are learning to talk, walk, communicate their needs, and regulate their emotions. They are exploring a whole new world in just a few short years!

Many studies show that a father's involvement and love in the initial years significantly affect a child's mental well-being, cognitive capabilities, resilience, maturity and patience, worldview, and sense of self (Ellis et al., 2017).

When dads care and play with the baby, when babies are still infants and toddlers, babies grow up to have fewer mental issues, better behavior, and advanced language development (Yogman & Garfield, 2016).

This means their social, emotional, and intellectual capabilities can flourish or suffer depending on the presence of a loving and attached relationship with their parents—with the critical role of dad.

If that wasn't surprising enough, even our simple gestures, like making eye contact with them, can influence how they communicate and bond with us (Leong et al., 2017). Hey, we all have seen those adorable videos where babies go crazy happy when parents look into the baby's eyes and engage comically, right?

Since that's the case, it's worth finding as many ways as possible to carve out extra free time during those first few hectic weeks. Trust me, you will need that time.

GETTING MORE TIME AND ENERGY ON YOUR AVERAGE DAY

The Doorbell Is Not Your Friend

Having relatives at your house as helpers is good, but not as guests! It would be best to limit visitors for the first few weeks or at least the first week. It's totally a good idea to put a sign that says "We are sleeping" or something similar when you or the baby is catching some z's.

Trust me, you don't want Aunt Mary barging in while you and your baby are trying to catch up on some much-needed sleep.

Storing Some Food

Make sure to have a stash of food that even the most sleep-deprived new dad can handle. Think of easy-to-prepare meals that require minimal effort.

You can do bulk cooking and freeze meals for the first few weeks. For some variety, you can use foods that can be eaten right after pan-heating them. Also, turn the meal leftovers into the next day's dish: Steak leftovers at dinner can become steak and eggs at breakfast, grilled chicken with salad turns into fajitas the next night, and so on. This helps the cooked meals go further.

And hey, don't be shy about serving these meals to guests or even treating yourself to them. After all, survival mode calls for culinary shortcuts!

Get More Sleep Like a Pro

Hey there, new dad. Let's talk about the art of surviving on minimal sleep. Brace yourself for those baby interruptions in the middle of the night, because they are about to become your routine. Sleeping a full night may feel like a distant dream, but there is no need to fear!

Sleep is a basic need, so let's make functioning on limited z's your new routine! Embrace the power of napping in the afternoon, and don't hesitate to call in reinforcements from your partner when you need a little extra shut-eye.

Tip:

Taking multiple 20–30-minute short naps throughout the day can often keep you going on less sleep. If you are a part of the 5 a.m. club, micro naps of 15 minutes after a morning workout and shower can help immensely. Additionally, it would help to take a nap after an afternoon meal, siesta style, to get a quick recharge.

Have the List of Priorities Ready

The goals and priorities list you set will help you get more time to

- get sleep
- bond with family
- handle household chores
- do personal development
- de-stress yourself

Now, let's look at what an essential baby kit looks like.

ESSENTIAL KIT FOR BABIES

Alright, new dads, let's talk about that baby kit before your little one arrives. You have to shop for things anyway, so why not get it done during the second trimester? Mom is feeling her best, you already know the baby's gender, and you don't have to stress about early labor signs like in the third trimester.

Now, I can't bore you with specific brand recommendations, but I will give you a list of the essentials. And hey, researching and becoming a baby product pro before the blurry days turn your mind into mush? That's pretty empowering, don't you think?

First-Aid Kit

Just like you have a kit for essential medicines in your home, you need a baby first-aid kit. Your baby first-aid kit should be like a trusty sidekick, ready to save the day. It needs to be portable, waterproof, and packed with all the superhero items you will need:

- **Painkillers:** Something like Ibuprofen can help infants (older than 2 months) with headaches and flu. If the baby gets a fever earlier, *go to a pediatrician.*

- **Bandages:** Your baby can get minor wounds or cuts when they wiggle around or crawl (roughly 6 months old). Bandages, along with an antiseptic ointment, can help you with that.

- **Calamine lotion:** We need something to deal with skin rashes, sunburns, and allergies.

- **Gas Drops:** In case the baby becomes particularly fussy after feeding.

- **Petroleum jelly:** For skin dryness and itchiness.

- **Ice packs:** Helps with relieving swelling and bumps.

- **Digital thermometer:** Putting a thermometer under your child's armpit can tell a quick result whether there's a fever or not.

Note:

Remember to check those sneaky expiry dates on your baby's medicines. You don't want to give them a dose of an expired drug accidentally! And hey, if your relatives or a babysitter are lending a helping hand, ensure they know where the first-aid kit is—just in case they need to perform some baby-saving heroics. If you think they might need extra guidance, throw in a first-aid manual, too. It's like an instruction manual but for tiny humans!

Accessories

- **Baby nail clippers:** The only requirement is safety.

- **Nasal suction device:** Helps you clean the baby's nasal passage.

If breastfeeding

- **Breast pump:** Electric ones are usually faster.

- **Nursing pillow:** Very much recommended as it helps your partner with posture.

Not Breastfeeding

- **Bottle and formula:** The only thing to keep in mind with baby bottles is to keep them clean and not use hours-old milk.

STOCKING THE BABY GEAR

Baby Clothes

Baby clothes remain the ultimate investment for new dads. We have onesies, rompers, sleepers, socks, mittens, hats, blankets, burp cloths, and more. Now, when it comes to investing, we know that a good amount is always better, right? Well, the same goes for those adorable onesies and rompers!

Trust me, you will be changing them multiple times in a day. So, get ready to either stock up on a bunch of them or become best friends with your laundry machine.

Diapers, Wipes, and Diaper Bag

Here's a tip to keep your diaper game strong: Stock up on diapers and wipes that can last a few weeks. And when the stock is empty, save yourself the hassle and order more online.

If you feel fancy and have an extra budget, why not treat yourself to a diaper bag? It's like a magical Mary Poppins bag that can fit everything from diapers to feeders. Whether on the go or chilling at home with the baby, having everything in one place will make your life much easier!

Car Seat, Stroller, and Baby Carrier

Having a baby car seat can save the day in so many ways. Whether taking them to visit relatives or just for a joyride, these seats keep your little one securely in place.

If you can, go for a convertible car seat that can grow with your baby from infancy to toddlerhood. They are like the transformers of car seats—adjusting to face backward when your baby is tiny and forward when the baby gets a little bigger.

Along with that, there are the strollers. They are like the wheels of parenthood, helping you transport your baby from home to car, from car to the shop, or even just for a stroll around the neighborhood in the morning.

Again, if you feel fancy and have extra funds, a baby carrier is a stylish accessory that brings you and your baby closer. It's like having a cuddle session while you go for walks.

Crib or Bassinet

They are both baby beds. You can buy both if you have the budget, but a crib is good enough otherwise.

A bassinet is more lightweight and can make breastfeeding easier, roughly up to the first 3 months. After that, you will still need a crib. So, see what your budget allows. Just remember, babies have a way of making you spend money on all sorts of things, so save where you can!

Life-Saving Toys

When buying toys for your little one, remember to keep your budget in mind. Babies are naturally curious, so they will enjoy playing with almost anything. But if you want to keep them entertained for extended periods, look for bite-friendly toys that offer different play styles.

Particularly, rubber toys can keep them engaged for anywhere from a few minutes to hours with minimal effort from you.

Here's another handy toy to keep your child busy: Find something that rattles when it's moved. It could be the classic set of keys (make sure they are made of nontoxic materials, don't have sharp edges, and no small parts) or a simple toy that produces sound (e.g., jiggling sound or music). The rattling noise will capture their attention and keep them happily occupied.

Rocking Chair

Kids love swinging. Something simple, like a rocking chair, can be a mighty helper. You see, babies can get a little fussy when they are tired, and that's where this magical chair comes in.

Believe it or not, it's like a sleep-inducing superpower! Just a few gentle rocks and your little one drifts off to dreamland, giving you and your partner much-needed shut-eye. And if the rocking chair has some gentle noisemaking things attached, it's a total win!

Baby-proofing Supplies

Hey, new dads, it's never too early to baby-proof your house. Trust me, those little bundles have a knack for rolling around and magically changing positions in the blink of an eye.

One minute, they are on their back; the next, they are on their tummy, and you are left wondering how they pulled off that feat! But wait, it gets even more exciting when they start crawling or attempting to stand up after 6 months. Suddenly, electric sockets and sharp furniture corners become the ultimate villains in your home.

So, my advice? Don't wait until your baby arrives or starts exploring their newfound mobility. Get ahead of the game and babyproof your house before the chaos!

Pacifier

One of the most touching moments as a dad is when you become a master at calming the crying baby. Having pacifiers is like having the cheat code of parenthood. These little wonders may look like feeder nipples, but they are way safer. Unlike regular nipples, pacifiers don't have any plastic that the baby can bite off and accidentally swallow. Trust me, you don't want those tiny plastic bits causing trouble inside your little one!

Whether on a road trip, a plane ride, or simply craving peace, the pacifier is your secret weapon to achieving that much-needed silence.

Note: Keep the pacifier clean: Don't put sweet things or honey (serious emphasis on no honey) on it, don't use it all the time, and don't attach it to a string. We don't want to put anything near the baby that they can get caught around their neck. Also, picking a one-piece pacifier as a two-piece pacifier can pose a choking risk if it breaks.

Baby Utensils and High Chair

Hey Dad, those small cups, containers, spoons, bowls, and bibs are your secret weapons against messiness.

They make feeding time a whole lot cleaner and more manageable. And when your little one starts devouring solids around 6 months, a high chair becomes your next best friend. It's like a mini throne for your baby's royal feasts.

Baby Bathtub

Let's dive into the world of bath time because it's so important that it can't be left out. Now, some dads worry a bit too much about bath time. For them, a baby bathtub is here to save the day.

With just 2 in. of water and a size that even the most clueless dad can handle, it behaves like a mini oasis for your little one. And hey, if you are feeling adventurous, you can always go for the regular bathtub option. Just remember to steer clear of the sink unless you want your baby to think they are a giant duck!

Now, can't we clean the baby with wipes and call it a day? Well, yes and no. While wipes and fresh clothes do wonders for keeping their skin clean, it's important to give babies proper baths, too.

However, it's essential to not go overboard with the bath sessions. Give your little one a break of about 2 days between each bath. Trust me, if you bathe them too much, their skin might feel drier than a desert, and you will need to use skin creams (and reduce baths). So, find that sweet spot and keep those baby bums squeaky clean!

Baby Monitoring

Now, when it comes to keeping an eye on your little one, you want some security that won't make your wallet cry.

Audio monitors that alert you and your partner when a baby makes noise can serve the basic needs. And for dads ready to take it up a notch, why not go for the ultimate security upgrade with a video monitor? You will have peace of mind and a front-row seat to all the cute and funny moments your baby has to offer. Who needs Netflix when you have your little show?

SOME OTHER THINGS ON THE CHECKLIST

A Change of Everything

Picture this: You are out, enjoying a nice meal at a restaurant or cruising in your car, when suddenly your little one decides it's the perfect time for a poop explosion. Trust me, it happens!

That's why it's crucial to always have a fully stocked baby essential kit on hand. Ensure you have everything, from diapers and spare clothes to wet wipes and feeders. Being prepared means you can easily handle messy situations, even in the most unexpected places. So, remember, keep that baby kit well-stocked!

Minding the Weather Forecast

It's time for you to become a weather expert! Always keep an eye on the forecast for rain and other weather conditions.

Remember, it's not just you and your partner on your adventures anymore. Mother Nature might just have a surprise in store, ready to rain on your parade! Hey, packing some adorable weatherproof clothes for your little one may do the trick.

Keep Stock of Snacks

Never be short of something for babies to chew or feed on, whether you are at home or traveling. If you forget that, things can quickly go from *feeling great* to *sanity on the verge of extinction* in no time!

Some Books

A good read for even 10 minutes can provide a timely respite. Additionally, if you read aloud, the baby may listen for a little while and possibly quiet down for 30 seconds!

Headphones

Dealing with that shrill cry for what feels like an eternity can push anyone's mind to the edge. But fear not, I have a solution that will make you relaxed in no time.

Picture this: You, rocking your baby to sleep, sporting a pair of stylish headphones. Not only will you protect your precious ears, but you will also get to enjoy some sweet music or catch up on your favorite podcast while tending to your little one. It's a win–win situation! Remember, breaks like that are okay if they help your sanity.

Cold, Flu, and Other Medicines

Hey, stock up on some medicines for yourself and your partner. Trust me, navigating the 1st year of parenthood can be a bit of a challenge, and it's even tougher when you both are feeling under the weather.

So, prepare those essential headache, stomach, and fever medicines, and take them when needed. You will need all your strength to keep up with your little bundle!

Health Insurance

Don't forget about insurance... for yourself! You are the superhero of the family, but even superheroes need a backup plan.

We don't want to leave the baby and mother without financial support in case something unexpected happens. Insurance can be that much-needed safety net to save the day!

Your Sense of Humor

Take things with a grain of salt. Remember, being a new dad means embracing the unexpected.

Your carefully laid-out plans for trips, work, and other activities will often need adjustments. So, go with the flow, keep a positive attitude, and don't forget to smile... a lot! Now, let's dive into what to do from day 1!

CONNECTING WITH THE BABY: STARTING FROM THE FIRST DAY

When you finally escape the hospital with the tiny human, don't be fooled by their pint-sized cuteness! These little ones have a knack for growing faster than weeds. So, buckle up. It's time to connect with your mini-me during these precious early years. Before you know it, that burrito will transform into a full-blown superhero ready to take on the world.

What to Do on the First Day and the First Week

The first and the next few days are the time to dive headfirst into the world of all things baby. Master the art of diaper changes and feeding, and become a pro with those wipes. And here's a tip: Don't be afraid to ask for help! Trust me, it's better to learn the ropes sooner rather than later. So, make it your primary mission to focus on these baby basics and build a rough routine. Remember, you have got this!

Skin-To-Skin Contact

Skin-to-skin contact is one of the best bonding methods in the first few days. There's just something about carrying the newborn that soothes the baby and the dad.

It's like a way to say hello and introduce yourself. Plus, the research side says that babies' vital signs stabilize through that contact. Just imagine, you get to officially say hello to your little one and have some relaxation time together (Shorey et al., 2016). It's a win–win!

Now, there's a particular type of skin-to-skin contact called kangaroo care. This is when you let your baby's bare chest rest on top of your bare chest. It's like having your own little kangaroo pouch! Research suggests that doing this for 1–2 hours daily is even better for your baby (Cleveland Clinic, 2023b). But remember, don't let the baby fall asleep in that position for too long. The baby should sleep on their back as a general rule.

And guess what? Skin-to-skin contact will remain one of the best playtimes for years to come. So, get ready for some great bonding moments with your little one!

Note:

Don't do this when you are sick, have used strong perfumes, or have smoked. Also, ensure the baby remains warm—you can use blankets, socks, and hats.

Tummy Time

Laying your baby's tummy down on the floor and watching them wiggle like crazy is like the first play with your baby! You are literally giving them a whole new perspective on the world!

Remember, use a soft and comfortably warm floor for this epic playtime. Doctors recommend tummy time because it helps strengthen the baby's back, neck, and arm muscles. It's like a baby boot camp for early crawling and early walking!

But hey, let's not forget essential tips for tummy time. Remember, the best sleeping and resting position is still on their back. Tummy time is just a fun little intermission from that. Start with short sessions of 3–5 minutes, 2–3 times a day, during the first few weeks. The goal is to gradually increase it to a whopping 20 minutes daily. Now, here are a few things to keep in mind:

- Stop when the baby starts getting quite fuzzy.

- Roll a small towel to prop their chest if their posture is wrong and their face is literally on the ground most of the time.

- Don't go away and leave the baby alone even for a few tens of seconds, as the baby may find it difficult to get oxygen if their head remains on the floor.

At 6 months, your baby will start to crawl or approach 1 hour of tummy time. It's a race between their mobility and love for belly-down relaxation!

Tip:

Kangaroo care we mentioned serves as its alternative.

BATHING THE BABY

The First Two Weeks

Changing diapers and using wet wipes on the face, neck, and diaper area is usually enough to keep your little one clean. But hey, we still need to give them a proper cleaning every 2 to 3 days.

Now, a gentle sponge bath is better for the first 2 weeks. Grab a sponge or washcloth and thoroughly clean your baby's skin—don't forget the armpits, chin, and behind the ears. It's like giving them a mini pampering session!

After Two Weeks

After 2 weeks, it's time to level up and move to the real deal in the bathtub. First, test if the water is warm, around 99 °F, before putting the baby in. You don't want your little one turning into a popsicle or spontaneously combusting. The water level should be about 2 in. high.

Posture: A safe posture when washing the baby is to support the baby's neck, head, and some upper back with one hand (non-dominant one) and clean with water using the other hand.

Note:

Don't give a bath right after meal time.

Feeding the Baby

Babies are milkaholics. They thrive on milk alone until they are around 4 months old. Yep, there's no need to (and you shouldn't) offer them anything else, not even a sip of water.

But once they hit the 4-month milestone, it's time to consult a pediatrician for some baby food advice. These experts will peek at your little one's health and weight and dish out some tasty recommendations on what and when to feed them.

Burping

Well, dad needs to take responsibility and burp the baby after feeding them, no? Burping the baby can be a very satisfying experience. It's a skill that will help the baby digest things and make you the envy of all the other dads at the playground.

So, embrace the art of baby burping, and watch as your little one becomes content for a few moments.

Posture: You can go with the good old posture: Baby's chin resting on the shoulder, one hand supporting the baby's neck and head, and the other lightly patting and rubbing the back. You can even rock the baby a little as the finishing touch.

PLAYING WITH THE BABY: FROM INFANTHOOD TO TODDLERHOOD

Helping with childcare is your secret gate to unlock a treasure trove of activities with your little one. Even in the first few days, you can wiggle their tiny hands, play peekaboo, and carry the boss baby around.

Learn to Love the Carrier and Stroller

Strollers and baby carriers are great for added safety in walking around and transporting the baby. A baby carrier allows you to carry your baby attached to your chest, while a stroller provides a car-like experience for them.

You Will See Many Different Shades of Poo

So, when playing with the little one, you will witness the incredible diversity of bodily excretions that tiny humans can produce. It's perplexing, really. How can something so adorable create something so... out of the world in smell? But hey, that's just part of the adventure! Below are some of the things you will see.

We want to avoid poop, but as new dads, poop knowledge should now be part of our dad repertoire. Baby poop and weight give us clues about how our little one is doing.

Breastfed babies have looser poop than formula-fed ones, as the baby can digest mom's milk with little leftovers. Formula-fed babies can have a paste-like stool similar to peanut butter's texture—but not firmer than that.

Now, don't panic if your baby loses a little weight (about 5%) in the first week or so (American Pregnancy Association, n.d.). However, if they continue losing weight or don't gain any at the rate recommended by a pediatrician after that period, it's time to call in the pediatrician. Here are a few more reasons to call the pediatrician (Chertoff, 2018a, 2018b):

- from the first 4 days, until the baby starts eating solids, the stool is any color other than greenish-yellow, yellow, brown, and yellowish-brown. Like black, red, green, or other colors—yes, more are possible

- unusual frequency of watery stools that seem like a case of diarrhea

- constipation in which the baby passes hard stool or shows pain when passing stool; the strain can even result in blood

- more stool than normal for your baby

- stool with an unusual amount of mucus or water

Distracting a Baby When There's No Boob for Feeding

You will get cried at... a lot! As new parents, all three of you will be experiencing a whirlwind of emotions, but the baby will be the most vocal about it.

Your role as a dad is to be there for Mom and provide support in childcare. As for the little one, you must unleash your bag of tricks! Carrying the baby, pulling hilarious faces, singing out off-key lullabies, spinning captivating stories, rocking them gently, and other creative methods are all on the table.

Using Different Holding Postures

Want to stop the baby from crying? Trying out different holding postures can help you silence that crying for a good 5 minutes (or more!).

- **Snuggle hold:** The head rests against the chest, one hand supports the neck, the other supports the butt, and the head is turned on one side. They can listen to your heartbeat if you put them on the left side.

- **Belly hold:** Baby's chest and belly drape over your forearm, your forearm close to your chest. Their head is toward the ground and back toward you. A little back tapping and rocking often work for any fuzzy baby!

- **Cradle hold:** Copy what the mom does: Support the head and neck with one arm and the butt with the other, and put the baby in the position of breastfeeding. It's a very natural posture. The catch is that the baby can start sucking and find out they have been defrauded!

Baby Sick Isn't So Bad

So, you are all prepared with a burp cloth (or some other cloth) draped over your shoulder, looking like a pro dad. But uh-oh! Out of nowhere, a splash of baby vomit lands on your neck.

Cue the panic, right? Wrong! Instead, think of it as your little one couldn't hold onto the milk for too long, and it's just a harmless milk splash. See? It's not so bad after all. Just clean it using a wet wipe.

Watch Those Hands

When you are with your baby, watch their little hands. Trust me, it's almost guaranteed that they will try to munch on something less than appetizing.

Whether it's an adventurous ant on the floor or a sneaky piece of garbage that somehow found its way into their tiny hands, it may end up in their tummy! So, stay vigilant and be ready!

Playing With Toys

Babies love to chew, and they love to use their hands and legs. As we previously discussed, toys that rattle, squeeze, and/or make noise are always a go to choice. They are great for helping them to learn, while giving dad face time with the little one.

Putting the Baby to Sleep

Putting the baby to sleep is like solving a Rubik's Cube—it's challenging but very satisfying! Now, it's mom who usually takes on this heroic task, but hey, don't let that stop you from getting in on the action! Research has our backs on this one, folks.

Turns out, when dads get involved in childcare, it can be a win–win for everyone involved. When fathers get involved with childcare and sometimes help in putting the baby to sleep, it can reduce the baby's urge to breastfeed, making them less wakeful, resulting in longer sleep for both Mom and Baby (Tikotzky et al., 2011).

So, the next time your little one decides to have a midnight party, try cradling them in a position similar to breastfeeding. They will be snoozing away in no time (unless they are super hangry, of course!).

Swaddling

This is an excellent trick to lull your little one into dreamland in the first few months. We can call it the "baby burrito" technique. You must wrap your baby snugly in a thin blanket, like a burrito!

It's done to recreate the cozy, snug environment they experienced in the womb. The baby feels all safe and secure, just like a warm hug from a fluffy cloud. And voila! The magic of security and warmth helps them drift into a peaceful slumber.

Note:

Remove the blanket when the baby tries to roll over, as that can be dangerous.

Get in the Car

When you feel like you are losing your mind from all the crying in the middle of the night, it may be time to take your baby for a joyride in your trusty vehicle.

If you have ever experienced the bliss of a long, comfortable road trip, you will know exactly what's about to happen to your little one. It's truly magical how the gentle hum of the engine can work its sleepy wonders. Just make sure to keep your baby cozy and warm!

Take Them Swimming

If you have the time and budget, consider enrolling your baby in a swimming class. Believe it or not, babies as young as 6 months old can learn to swim with proper supervision. They may even outswim their dad!

Swimming can be tiring and fun for kids, so you may get extra sleep. Also, who knows? Maybe your little one will become the next Michael Phelps!

Spend Some Quiet Time

Sitting still and watching your baby play and wiggle around can be surprisingly stress-relieving. It's like a mini show, except the star is a tiny human who can't talk yet! You may even get 2 minutes of pure joy before they decide it's time to crank up the volume and start crying again!

So, new dad, that's the all-rounder guide to the first few months after birth. Playing with the baby and creating a bond with them when they are a newborn (less than 1 month old) and infant (greater than 1 month old) is very important. There are many ways to play with the baby, but you should remember the safety tips when playing with them. Also, you should continue to increase your knowledge about the baby's development milestones to do conscious parenting. Now, the next chapter will conclude this journey, and set the stage for the next one to begin!

Notes

PREGNANCY GUIDE FOR FIRST-TIME DADS

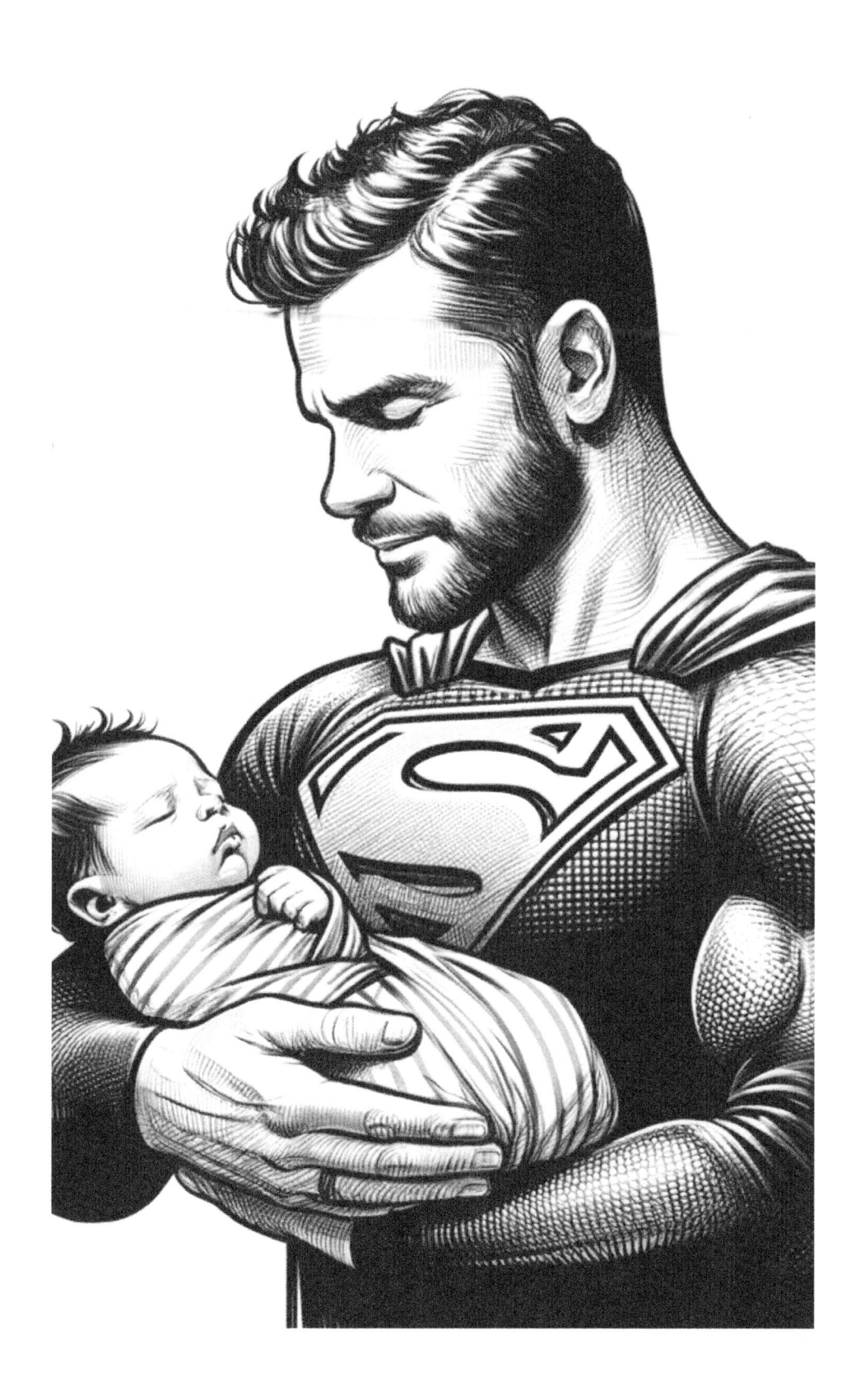

Conclusion

If you've made it this far into the book, congratulations! You have officially survived the equivalent of a crash course in biology, psychology, and a few other -ologies that I may have invented along the way. You've traversed the complex world of diaper sizes, learned to sympathize with morning sickness, grappled with your fears and anxieties, juggled societal expectations, and started forming a bond with a being that, at this point, you've probably only seen as a cute, blurry ultrasound photo.

This book's primary aim was to walk you through this crazy, beautiful journey from a bun-in-the-oven to a baby-in-your-arms. To prepare you, my fellow first-time fathers, for the rollercoaster that awaits and reassure you that it's okay to scream a little, or a lot.

Understanding Pregnancy was about demystifying the miracle of life, charting the changes that occur stage by stage. I assure you, you will never look at a melon (or any fruit for that matter) the same way again!

As *The Supportive Partner*, you've grasped the importance of being the rock when the hormones hit the fan, learning the art of foot rubs, and mastering the correct response to "Do I look fat in this?"

Mental and Emotional Well-being was all about dealing with your fears and anxieties. Don't forget, it's okay to freak out a bit - just remember to use your 'inside voice.'

Navigating Social Pressures and Expectations taught us the delicate art of juggling societal expectations, work pressures, and our own aspirations of fatherhood. It's like spinning plates while riding a unicycle. But trust me, with a little practice and a few faceplants, you'll get the hang of it.

Bonding with the Baby highlighted the joy and significance of creating an early bond with your baby. And let's face it, any excuse to talk to the belly without seeming crazy is a win!

Now, my brave first-time dads, it's time for you to take this treasure trove of knowledge, tips, and dad-jokes and embark on your unique journey of fatherhood. Remember, every pregnancy, every baby, every father is different. And that's okay. In fact, it's more than okay, it's beautiful.

Throughout this journey, continue learning, growing, and laughing at the absurdity that sometimes accompanies fatherhood. Share your experiences with other first-time fathers and create a community where support, wisdom, and more dad-jokes can be exchanged freely.

In the end, remember this - while pregnancy and fatherhood might throw you into a world of unknowns, a world that can sometimes feel challenging, confusing, or even overwhelming, it's also a world filled with immense love, joy, and fulfilment. You're not alone in this journey. You're stepping into a global fraternity of fathers who, just like you, are trying their best, making some mistakes, but ultimately loving their little ones with all they've got.

So here's to you, soon-to-be dad. May your dad-jokes always be groan-worthy, your shoulders strong for piggybacks, and your heart full of the incredible love that comes with being a father. Here's to the greatest adventure of your life. You've got this! Happy parenting First-Time Dads!

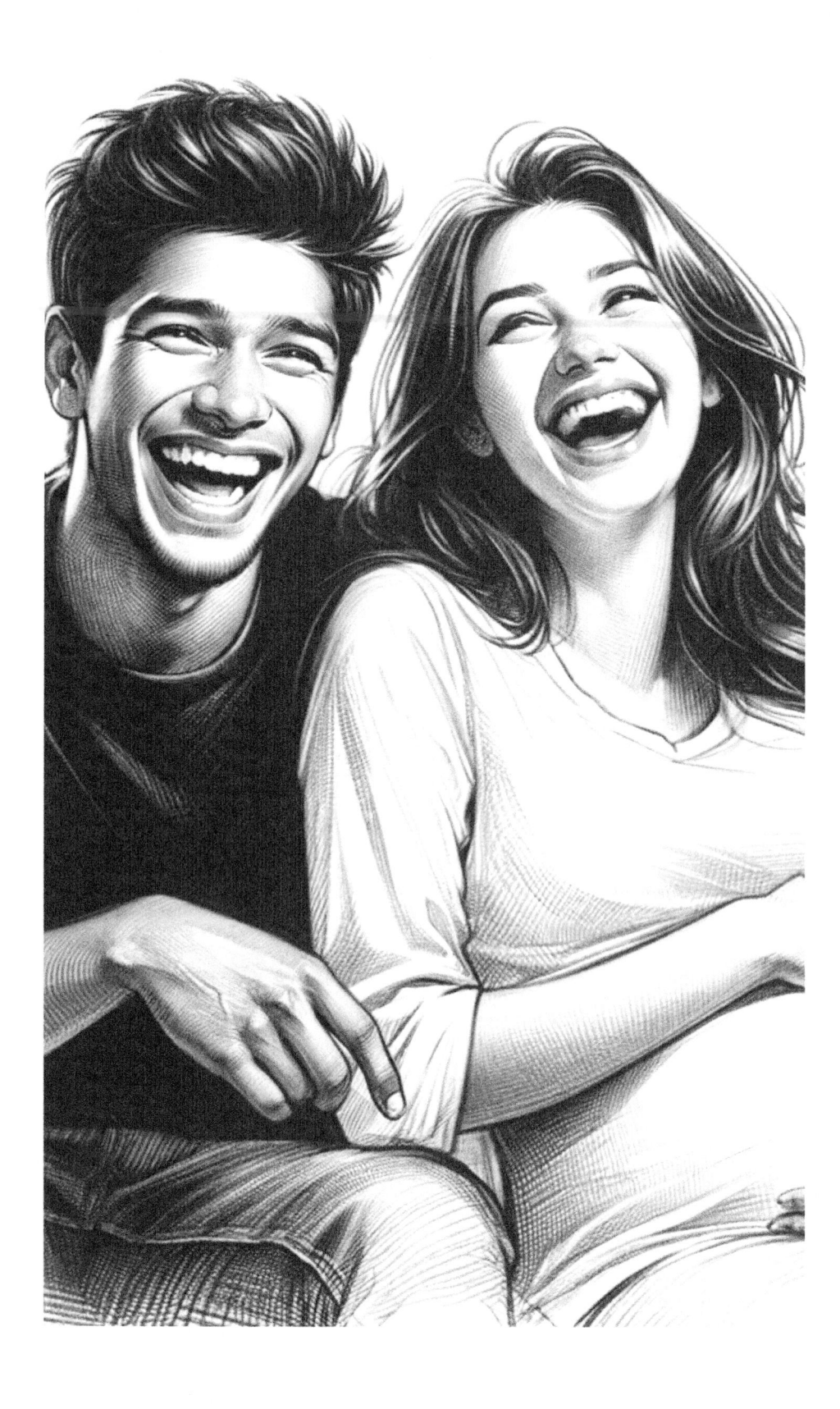

Afterword

As I sit to write this afterword, the echoes of laughter from my two young boys dance through the halls of our home. Their joyous cacophony, a testament to the journey of fatherhood, is a melody that resonates deep within me. I, Taylor Anthony, am not just an author, but a father, a husband, and a student of life, learning from the tiniest teachers - my sons.

Parenthood, I've realized, is a voyage through the seasons of time. It begins as a whisper, a faint heartbeat inside a womb, growing into a crescendo of life that transforms us in ways we never imagined. From the first time you hear that heartbeat, to the magical moment when you hold your child for the first time, each second is a brushstroke on the canvas of your heart.

Fatherhood is not just a role; it is an evolution. In the early days, time feels like a relentless river, rushing past as you traverse sleepless nights, first steps, and uncharted worries. But in those moments, amongst the chaos and coffee cups, you find the true essence of love - unconditional and infinite.

As your child grows, so do you. Each day brings a new chapter, a fresh challenge, and a different joy. Watching them discover the world, with wide-eyed wonder and boundless curiosity, is a reminder of life's simplest yet profound pleasures.

But with the joys come the trials. There will be times when you doubt yourself; when the weight of responsibility feels too heavy. In these moments, remember, the oak tree was once just a seed. Strength and wisdom come not from ease, but from weathering storms.

As you continue on this journey, know that the passage of time is relentless, but within its march lies beauty. The first words, the first bike ride, the first day of school - each a fleeting, precious moment. Cherish them. Embrace them. For in the blink of an eye, those tiny hands that once clung to yours will be strong enough to forge their own path.

And to you, the first-time dad reading this, let these words be your beacon. Love deeply, guide gently, and grow alongside your child. Your journey will be unique, filled with its own stories and songs. Trust in yourself, in the love you possess, and in the journey you are on.

Parenthood is the grandest adventure of all. It is a journey not measured in years, but in moments - moments that fill your heart and soul with an indescribable love. Embrace each day, for these days, are the fabric that weaves the patchwork quilt of your life.

In closing, remember this - you are not just raising a child; you are raising the future. And in your hands, with love, patience, and wisdom, lies the power to shape a life, a destiny, and a legacy.

With warmth and understanding,

Taylor Anthony

Glossary

A

Afterbirth: Placenta and membranes delivered after the baby.

Afterpains: Cramps after birth as uterus shrinks.

Alpha-Fetoprotein Screening (AFP): Blood test for birth defects.

Amniotic Fluid: Water-like fluid surrounding the baby in the womb.

B

Basal Body Temperature: Body temperature at rest; used for fertility tracking.

Biophysical Profile: Ultrasound assessing baby's health.

Birth Plan: Plan for labor and delivery preferences.

Bloody Show: Discharge signifying labor is near.

Braxton Hicks: False, irregular contractions; not real labor.

PREGNANCY GUIDE FOR FIRST-TIME DADS

Breech Position: Baby positioned bottom or feet first.

C

Cervix: Lower part of the uterus, opens during birth.

Cesarean Section (C-Section): Surgical birth of the baby.

Chorionic Villus Sampling (CVS): Test for genetic disorders.

Colostrum: Early breast milk, rich in nutrients.

Conception: When sperm meets egg.

Contractions: Uterus muscles tightening for childbirth.

Crowning: Baby's head starting to emerge during birth.

D

Dilation: Opening of the cervix for childbirth.

Doula: Non-medical person assisting with childbirth.

E

Eclampsia: Serious high blood pressure in pregnancy.

Ectopic Pregnancy: Pregnancy outside the uterus.

Edema: Swelling, often in feet and ankles.

Effacement: Thinning of the cervix for birth.

Embryo: Baby's earliest development stage.

Engagement: Baby's head moving into position for birth.

Epidural: Pain relief injection in the spine during labor.

F

Fetus: Term for baby after eight weeks of development.

Folic Acid: Vitamin important for fetal development.

Fontanelles: Soft spots on baby's head.

Fundal Height: Measurement from pubic bone to top of uterus.

G

Gestation: Duration of pregnancy.

Gestational Age: Baby's age in weeks since conception.

Gestational Diabetes: Diabetes developed during pregnancy.

Glucose Test: Checks for gestational diabetes.

Gravidity: Number of times a woman has been pregnant.

H

HCG (Human Chorionic Gonadotropin): Pregnancy hormone.

Heartburn: Burning sensation in chest, common in pregnancy.

Hormones: Chemicals in the body influencing pregnancy.

Hyperemesis Gravidarum: Severe nausea and vomiting.

I

Implantation: Fertilized egg attaching to the womb lining.

In Vitro Fertilization (IVF): Assisted reproductive technology.

Induction: Artificially starting labor.

Intrauterine Device (IUD): Contraceptive device.

Jaundice: Yellowing of baby's skin, often harmless.

K

Kegel Exercises: Exercises to strengthen pelvic floor muscles.

Kick Counts: Counting baby's movements in the womb.

L

Lactation Consultant: Breastfeeding expert.

Lactation: Production of breast milk.

Lamaze: Breathing method for labor pain management.

Lanugo: Fine hair covering newborn.

Linea Nigra: Dark line on the belly during pregnancy.

M

Meconium: Baby's first stool, usually passed after birth.

Midwife: Trained pregnancy and birth specialist.

Montgomery Glands: Glands on areola, enlarge during pregnancy.

Morning Sickness: Nausea during pregnancy.

Mucus Plug: Seals the cervix, dislodges before labor.

N

Nausea: Morning sickness, common in early pregnancy.

Nesting: Urge to prepare home for baby's arrival.

NICU (Neonatal Intensive Care Unit): Care unit for sick or premature babies.

Nonstress Test: Monitoring baby's heart rate

Nuchal Cord: Umbilical cord around baby's neck.

O

Obstetrician: Doctor specialized in pregnancy and childbirth.

Ovulation: Release of egg from ovary.

Oxytocin: Hormone stimulating labor contractions.

P

Perineum: Area between genitals and anus.

Pitocin: Synthetic oxytocin to induce labor.

Placenta: Organ providing oxygen and nutrients to the baby.

Postpartum: Period after childbirth.

Preeclampsia: Pregnancy complication with high blood pressure.

Q

Quickening: First felt movements of the baby.

R

Rh Factor: Determines compatibility of mother's and baby's blood types.

Rooming-in: Baby stays in the room with parents at the hospital.

Round Ligament Pain: Pain from stretching ligaments.

S

SIDS (Sudden Infant Death Syndrome): Unexplained death of a baby less than a year old.

Sonogram/Ultrasound: Image of the baby inside the womb.

Stretch Marks: Skin marks from stretching during pregnancy.

Surfactant: Substance helping baby's lungs function.

T

Teratogen: Anything causing birth defects.

Tocolytic: Medication to delay labor.

Trimester: One of three pregnancy stages, each about three months.

U

Umbilical Cord: Cord connecting baby to the placenta.

Uterus: Womb where the baby grows.

V

Vacuum Extraction: Assisted delivery method.

Varicose Veins: Swollen veins, common in pregnancy.

Vernix: Waxy coating protecting baby's skin in the womb.

W

Water Break: Rupture of amniotic sac, signaling labor.

Weaning: Transitioning baby from breast milk/formula to solid foods.

X

X-Ray: Generally avoided during pregnancy.

Y

Yeast Infection: Common infection during pregnancy.

Yolk Sac: Early source of nutrients for the embryo.

Z

Zinc: Important mineral for pregnancy health.

Zygote: The fertilized egg in the first days post-conception.

References

Allen, S., & Daly, K. (2007). *The effects of father involvement: An updated research summary of the evidence.* Father Involvement Research Alliance. https://www.fatherhood.gov/sites/default/files/resource_files/effects_of_father_involvement.pdf

American College of Obstetricians and Gynecologists. (n.d.). *Exercise during pregnancy.* https://www.acog.org/womens-health/faqs/exercise-during-pregnancy

American Pregnancy Association. (n.d.). *Newborn weight gain.* https://americanpregnancy.org/healthy-pregnancy/first-year-of-life/newborn-weight-gain/

Barth, L. (2023, October 16). *Pregnancy mood swings: Why you're feeling them and what to do.* Healthline. https://www.healthline.com/health/pregnancy/pregnancy-mood-swings#pregnancy-sign

Bjarnadottir, A. (2023, June 2). *13 foods to eat when you're pregnant.* Healthline. https://www.healthline.com/nutrition/13-foods-to-eat-when-pregnant

Bradley, S. (2020, May 7). *Baby blues: How long they last and what you can do*. Healthline. https://www.healthline.com/health/baby-blues#symptoms

Bustos, M., Venkataramanan, R., & Caritis, S. (2016, May 13). Nausea and vomiting of pregnancy - What's new? *Autonomic Neuroscience: Basic & Clinical, 202*, 62–72. https://doi.org/10.1016/j.autneu.2016.05.002

Cherney, K. (2023, July 3). *Baby poop: What's typical and when to see a pediatrician*. Healthline. https://www.healthline.com/health/parenting/baby-poop-color#poop-color-and-health

Chertoff, J. (2018a, October 1). *How often should a newborn poop?* Healthline. https://www.healthline.com/health/parenting/how-often-should-a-newborn-poop#by-age

Chertoff, J. (2018b, October 29). *Breastfed poop: Color, texture, frequency, smell, and more.* Healthline. https://www.healthline.com/health/parenting/breastfed-poop#seeking-help

Chi, E. (2019, August 26). *Morning sickness: Causes, treatments, and prevention. Healthline.* https://www.healthline.com/health/morning-sickness#tests

Cinelli, E. (2022, October 19). *Yoga poses to avoid during pregnancy.* Verywell Family. https://www.verywellfamily.com/yoga-poses-to-avoid-during-pregnancy-5181459

Cleveland Clinic. (2022, April 5). *What is a midwife? When to see one & what to expect.* https://my.clevelandclinic.org/health/articles/22648-midwife

Cleveland Clinic. (2023a, April 5). *Morning sickness: When it starts, treatment & prevention.* https://my.clevelandclinic.org/health/diseases/16566-morning-sickness-nausea-and-vomiting-of-pregnancy

Cleveland Clinic. (2023b, August 11). *Kangaroo care (Skin to skin): What it is & benefits.* https://my.clevelandclinic.org/health/treatments/12578-kangaroo-care

DaddiLife. (2018, March 9). *The new dad's survival guide: 101 tips for dads, by dads.* https://www.daddilife.com/family/expecting/first-time-dads/

Dingel, H., Rae, M., & Cox, C. (2022, July 13). *Health costs associated with pregnancy, childbirth, and postpartum care.* Peterson-KFF Health System Tracker. https://www.healthsystemtracker.org/brief/health-costs-associated-with-pregnancy-childbirth-and-postpartum-care/

Dix, M. (2019, October 23). *When does morning sickness start? Plus, how to manage it.* Healthline. https://www.healthline.com/health/pregnancy/when-does-morning-sickness-start#treatment

Ellis, S. M., Khan, Y. S., Harris, V. W., McWilliams, R., & Converse, D. (2017, September 18). *The impact of fathers on children's well-being.* IFAS Extension, University of Florida. https://edis.ifas.ufl.edu/publication/FY1451

Eunice Kennedy Shriver National Institute of Child Health and Human Development. (2017, January 31). *What happens during prenatal visits?* U.S. Department of Health and Human Services, National Institutes of Health. https://www.nichd.nih.gov/health/topics/preconceptioncare/conditioninfo/prenatal-visits

Hinkle, S. N., Mumford, S. L., Grantz, K. L., Silver, R. M., Mitchell, E. M., Sjaarda, L. A., Radin, R. G., Perkins, N. J., Galai, N., & Schisterman, E. F. (2016). Association of nausea and vomiting during pregnancy with pregnancy loss: a secondary analysis of a randomized clinical trial. *JAMA Internal Medicine, 176*(11), 1621–1627. https://doi.org/10.1001/jamainternmed.2016.5641

Hoekzema, E., Steenbergen, H. v., Straathof, M., Beekmans, A., Freund, I. M., Pouwels, P. J. W., & Crone, E. A. (2022, November 2). Mapping the effects of pregnancy on resting state brain activity, white matter microstructure, neural metabolite concentrations and grey matter architecture. *Nature Communications, 13*, Article 6931. https://doi.org/10.1038/s41467-022-33884-8

Holland, K. (2023, June 26). *Symptoms of pregnancy: 15 early signs you might notice.* Healthline. https://www.healthline.com/health/pregnancy/early-symptoms-timeline#symptoms

Hoyert, D. L. (2023, March 16). *Maternal mortality rates in the United States, 2021.* Centers for Disease Control and Prevention. https://www.cdc.gov/nchs/data/hestat/maternal-mortality/2021/maternal-mortality-rates-2021.htm

Ibrahim, M. H., Somers, J. A., Luecken, L. J., Fabricius, W. V., & Cookston, J. T. (2017). Father–adolescent engagement in shared activities: Effects on cortisol stress response in young adulthood. *Journal of Family Psychology, 31*(4), 485–494 https://doi.org/10.1037/fam0000259

Jirsaraie, R. J., Palma, A. M., Small, S. L., Sandman, C. A., Davis, E. P., Baram, T. Z., Stern, H., Glynn, L. M., & Yassa, M. A. (2023). Prenatal exposure to maternal mood entropy is associated with a weakened and inflexible salience network in adolescence. *Biological Psychiatry: Cognitive Neuroscience and Neuroimaging*, Article S2451-9022(23)00215-X. https://doi.org/10.1016/j.bpsc.2023.08.002

Kinsella, M. T., & Monk, C. (2009). Impact of maternal stress, depression and anxiety on fetal neurobehavioral development. *Clinical Obstetrics and Gynecology, 52*(3), 425–440 https://doi.org/10.1097/GRF.0b013e3181b52df1

Koessmeier, C., & Büttner, O. B. (2021). Why are we distracted by social media? Distraction situations and strategies, reasons for distraction, and individual differences. *Frontiers in Psychology, 12*, Article 711416. https://doi.org/10.3389/fpsyg.2021.711416

Kroenke, K., Spitzer, R. L., & Williams, J. B. (2001). The PHQ-9: Validity of a brief depression severity measure. *Journal of General Internal Medicine, 16*, 606–613. https://doi.org/10.1046/j.1525-1497.2001.016009606.x

Leong, V., Byrne, E., Clackson, K., Georgieva, S., Lam, S., & Wass, S. (2017). Speaker gaze increases information coupling between infant and adult brains. *Proceedings of the National*

Academy of Sciences, 114(50), 13290–13295.https://doi.org/10.1073/pnas.1702493114

Lindberg, S. (2020, February 19). *Weight gain in first trimester: How much is normal?* Healthline. https://www.healthline.com/health/pregnancy/weight-gain-first-trimester

Livingston, G., & Parker, K. (2019, June 12). *For father's day, 8 facts about American dads.* Pew Research Center. https://www.pewresearch.org/short-reads/2019/06/12/fathers-day-facts/

Machin, A. (2021, June 19). *In praise of fathers: The making of the modern dad.* The Guardian. https://www.theguardian.com/lifeandstyle/2021/jun/19/in-praise-of-fathers-the-making-of-the-modern-dad

Mandl, E. (2023, January 2). *The 14 best foods to eat when you're nauseous.* Healthline. https://www.healthline.com/nutrition/foods-to-eat-when-nauseous#10

March of Dimes. (n.d.-a). *Postpartum depression.* https://www.marchofdimes.org/find-support/topics/postpartum/postpartum-depression

March of Dimes. (n.d.-b). *Baby blues after pregnancy.* https://www.marchofdimes.org/find-support/topics/postpartum/baby-blues-after-pregnancy

Marcin, A. (2017, October 27). *Your week-by-week pregnancy calendar.* Healthline. https://www.healthline.com/health/pregnancy/week-by-week-calendar#Week-13

Marcin, A. (2023, July 21). *How to prevent stretch marks: 7 tips.* Healthline. https://www.healthline.com/health/how-to-prevent-stretch-marks#weight-control

Marnach, M. (2023, April 12). *Leg cramps during pregnancy: Preventable?* Mayo Clinic. https://www.mayoclinic.org/healthy-lifestyle/pregnancy-week-by-week/expert-answers/leg-cramps-during-pregnancy/faq-20057766

Mayo Clinic Staff. (2022a, February 8). *Preterm labor - Symptoms and causes.* Mayo Clinic. https://www.mayoclinic.org/diseases-conditions/preterm-labor/symptoms-causes/syc-20376842

Mayo Clinic Staff. (2022b, February 18). *Pregnancy diet: Focus on these essential nutrients.* Mayo Clinic. https://www.mayoclinic.org/healthy-lifestyle/pregnancy-week-by-week/in-depth/pregnancy-nutrition/art-20045082

Mayo Clinic Staff. (2022c, March 9). *3rd trimester pregnancy: What to expect.* Mayo Clinic. https://www.mayoclinic.org/healthy-lifestyle/pregnancy-week-by-week/in-depth/pregnancy/art-20046767

Mayo Clinic Staff. (2022d, April 09). *Gestational diabetes - Symptoms & causes.* Mayo Clinic. https://www.mayoclinic.org/diseases-conditions/gestational-diabetes/symptoms-causes/syc-20355339

Mayo Clinic Staff. (2022e, April 19). *Prenatal vitamins: Why they matter, how to choose.* Mayo Clinic. https://www.mayoclinic.org/healthy-lifestyle/pregnancy-week-by-week/in-depth/prenatal-vitamins/art-20046945

Mayo Clinic Staff. (2022f, August 06). *Prenatal care: 1st trimester visits*. Mayo Clinic. https://www.mayoclinic.org/healthy-lifestyle/pregnancy-week-by-week/in-depth/prenatal-care/art-20044882

Mayo Clinic Staff. (2022g, December 06). *High-risk pregnancy: Know what to expect*. Mayo Clinic. https://www.mayoclinic.org/healthy-lifestyle/pregnancy-week-by-week/in-depth/high-risk-pregnancy/art-20047012

Mayo Clinic Staff. (2023, March 10). *Zinc*. Mayo Clinic. https://www.mayoclinic.org/drugs-supplements-zinc/art-20366112

Metzger, G. K. (2022, August 9). *Pregnancy glossary*. WebMD. https://www.webmd.com/baby/pregnancy-glossary

Mridha, D. (n.d.). *Debasish Mridha quotes*. Goodreads. https://www.goodreads.com/quotes/7444656-fear-comes-from-the-lack-of-knowledge-and-a-state

Nall, R. (2018, September 5). *The third trimester of pregnancy: Pain and insomnia*. Healthline. https://www.healthline.com/health/pregnancy/third-trimester-pain-insomnia#insomnia-prevention

Office on Women's Health in the Office of the Assistant Secretary for Health. (2023, October 17). *Postpartum depression*. U.S. Department of Health & Human Services. https://www.womenshealth.gov/mental-health/mental-health-conditions/postpartum-depression

Peale, N. V. (n.d.). *Norman Vincent Peale quotes.* Goodreads. https://www.goodreads.com/quotes/4324-shoot-for-the-moon-even-if-you-miss-you-ll-land

Pietrangelo, A. (2022, March 31). *Postpartum depression: Symptoms, treatment, causes & more.* Healthline. https://www.healthline.com/health/depression/postpartum-depression#treatment

Pittman, F. (n.d.). *Frank Pittman quotes.* Goodreads. https://www.goodreads.com/quotes/286735-the-guys-who-fear-becoming-fathers-don-t-understand-that-fathering

Rasmussen, K. M., Catalano, P. M., & Yaktine, A. L. (2009). New guidelines for weight gain during pregnancy: What obstetrician/gynecologists should know. *Current Opinion in Obstetrics & Gynecology, 21*(6), 521–526. https://doi.org/10.1097/GCO.0b013e328332d24e

Rivelli, E. (2022, November 30). *Best health insurance options for pregnant women.* Forbes Advisor. https://www.forbes.com/advisor/health-insurance/health-insurance-for-pregnant-women/

Shorey, S., He, H. G., & Morelius, E. (2016). Skin-to-skin contact by fathers and the impact on infant and paternal outcomes: An integrative review. *Midwifery, 40,* 207–217. https://doi.org/10.1016/j.midw.2016.07.007

Social Work Blog NASW. (2016, December 8). *Expectant fathers' beliefs and expectations about fathering as they prepare to parent a new infant.* https://www.socialworkblog.org/nasw-press/journals-nasw-publications/2016/12/expectant-fathers-beliefs-and-expectations-about-fathering-as-they-prepare-to-parent-a-new-infant/

Stothart, C., Mitchum, A., & Yehnert, C. (2015). The attentional cost of receiving a cell phone notification. *Journal of Experimental Psychology: Human Perception and Performance, 41*(4), 893–897. https://doi.org/10.1037/xhp0000100

Tikotzky, L., Sadeh, A., & Glickman-Gavrieli, T. (2011). Infant sleep and paternal involvement in infant caregiving during the first 6 months of life. *Journal of Pediatric Psychology, 36*(1), 36–46. https://doi.org/10.1093/jpepsy/jsq036

Walsh, K. (2023, April 7). *Faces of healthcare: What's an OB-GYN?* Healthline. https://www.healthline.com/find-care/articles/obgyns/what-is-an-obgyn

Wang, Z.-W., Hua, J., & Xu, Y.-H. (2015, May 28). The relationship between gentle tactile stimulation on the fetus and its temperament 3 months after birth. *Behavioural Neurology, 2015*, Article 371906. https://doi.org/10.1155/2015/371906

Watson, S. (2023, March 22). *Third trimester of pregnancy: What to expect, fetal development.* WebMD. https://www.webmd.com/baby/third-trimester-of-pregnancy

WebMD Editorial Contributors. (2022, August 8). *Premature (preterm) labor: Signs, causes, and treatments*. WebMD. https://www.webmd.com/baby/premature-labor#1-2

Weishaupt, J. (2021, November 9). *Baby first aid kit essentials: What to include in the box?* WebMD. https://www.webmd.com/parenting/baby/what-to-put-in-baby-first-aid-kit

What to Expect Editors. (2021, November 16). *Pregnancy glossary: A to Z guide to pregnancy terminology*. What to Expect. https://www.whattoexpect.com/pregnancy/glossary

Yogman, M., & Garfield, C. F. (2016). Fathers' roles in the care and development of their children: The role of pediatricians. *Pediatrics*, *138*(1), Article e20161128. https://doi.org/10.1542/peds.2016-1128